Pregnancy:
The Ins and Outs,
Ups and Downs

Gracie Little

DEDICATION

This book is dedicated to my very own little monsters

With all my love and thanks for the ride so far

You know I love you, and you know who you are

CONTENTS

ACKNOWLEDGMENTS

Many thanks to my husband for putting up with us all. Thanks also to the kiddiewinks, without whom I wouldn't have any of the experiences I write about in this book.

My best wishes go to all hospital employees, especially the midwives, nurses and doctors of the NHS who mostly go unthanked for all the amazing work they do each and every day.

Even more good wishes go to all the women who are about to embark on this amazing adventure or who have already been through it. You are all amazing!

1 INTRODUCTION

You're pregnant! First and foremost CONGRATULATIONS! Pregnancy is one of the most exciting, emotional and tiring experiences you will ever live through – the second being the first year of your child's life! You will have more ups and downs than you ever imagined, and hopefully will start to bond with your baby before they even enter the world.

If you're wondering what makes me qualified to write a book about pregnancy, I have three children – all boys – though I have zero medical experience. I decided to write this book to provide a first-hand insight into pregnancy and all its ups and downs. I'm hoping that this book will help you learn what to look out for, give you an idea on what to expect from your pregnancy and get the ins and outs of what I experienced. Not for a second do I profess to have any kind of professional qualification, but I've been there and done that and even bought a t-shirt or two – mostly maternity ones.

Hopefully reading about how my pregnancies went will give you an idea of how yours may go, though each and every pregnancy will be different. Some things tend to run through the same, such as the ever-growing bump and constant tiredness in the first trimester, but you may experience vastly different symptoms or complaints or feelings. The best advice I can give is to enjoy your pregnancy, sure there's bits each of us dislike about it but it will soon all be over and believe it or not, you will get bump envy at some point!

Whilst I enjoyed aspects of my pregnancy there were definitely certain things I could have done without. The highlights make the low points worth it though.

For me, the number one highlight of pregnancy was feeling my baby kick. The number one downside was definitely the heartburn in the third trimester. But the highlights far outweighed the low points, and it all faded into the background once my baby was born.

You may think you won't be like every other pregnant woman and carry on regardless, but there will be points when you just can't do the things you used to do, such as painting your toenails in your seventh month of pregnancy! For me, I realised I was the stereotypical pregnant woman when I started repeatedly rubbing my bump whenever I got the chance. In the past it had always annoyed me how pregnant women couldn't keep their hands off their bellies, like they had to point out the obvious. I quickly learnt it was nothing to do with showing off and everything to do with a special kind of love. I even caught myself talking to my baby in the shower; again I was never going to be one of them.

I can't say what the highlights and low points will be for you as each and every pregnancy is different, and of course we are all different, but I can say that it will be a rollercoaster of a ride, and one that you will be ready to get off at the end. Though I can't promise that you won't want to get back on after a few months!

I'm pretty sure this doesn't apply to everyone but after moaning about feeling uncomfortable throughout my pregnancy, once I had my babies I'd always feel slightly envious of other pregnant women. Why? Because when you're pregnant you are a walking miracle, and you can't help but feel special and privileged to be bringing life into the world.

Enjoy your pregnancy. Yes sometimes you may wish you weren't, but for the majority of the time you'll love it. And believe me; you will get bump envy when it's gone – although you will have a beautiful baby in its place.

I hope you enjoy this book, and get something out of it, whether its advice, a piece of information you didn't know or a laugh and an "I have that" moment.

2 THE GETTING PREGNANT BIT

If you've picked up this book then chances are that you are already pregnant, but if you're still trying there are certain things you can do to help Mother Nature along the way.

First, have sex. Lots of it. If not for any other reason but to get it while you can…when your baby comes you'll be too tired!

Second, eat and drink healthily. If you want to get pregnant then your body needs to be ready for the hormonal changes it is going to face. Eating healthily increases your chances of getting pregnant, as does exercising and cutting down on alcohol and any other bad habits such as smoking.

Eating and drinking healthily is not just limited to you though. Your partner should also be cutting down as their sperm also needs to be in optimal condition. Tell them to put down that cigarette, throw away the burger and stay in rather than go to the pub. Okay, maybe none of that worked, but get them involved, show them the facts and if necessary take them along to your doctor with you if you go to discuss pregnancy.

Thirdly, start taking folic acid now. Your body needs extra folic acid for the baby and you can either buy simple folic acid capsules or pregnancy vitamins with added folic acid. Whilst your body will already store folic acid, it does not store a lot, and the benefits of taking it are well known. Basically, your body needs the folic acid to provide an optimal environment for your baby, and your baby needs it to grow, particularly in the first 3 months. You can even give yourself an extra dose by upping your intake of green vegetables such as broccoli, sprouts and spinach, all of which contain folic acid.

If you haven't already, inform your doctor of your decision to try and get pregnant. They may be able to offer advice that is more tailored to your specific needs and will be able to monitor your health and deal with any questions and worries you may have further down the line.

We touched on it briefly above, but the other main thing you should do if you want to get pregnant is to exercise. If you already have a good workout routine then maintain it. If you don't, get working on it. It is easier to get pregnant if your body is healthy and your pregnancy will run smoother if you can maintain some form of exercise throughout.

If, like me, you're not a fitness fanatic then try something more relaxing. Yoga or Pilates are both fantastic exercise classes and you should be able to find classes specifically for pregnancy and post-pregnancy stages.

Finally, try to cut out any stress or negativity in your life. You want to be as relaxed as you can while trying to get pregnant. It may be easier said than done of course, but taking time out is important. Whether your particular brand of relaxation is a relaxing bath or reading a good book snuggled up on the couch, do it, and do it often. This is not slouching; it is getting your body in optimum shape for your pregnancy.

So to summarise, to increase your chances of getting pregnant you need to do the following:

- ➢ Have regular sex
- ➢ It should go without saying that now would be a good time to stop any contraceptive methods you may have been trying
- ➢ Eat healthy
- ➢ Cut down on unhealthy habits, including drinking, smoking and any drugs
- ➢ Take folic acid, and other pregnancy vitamins if required
- ➢ Consult your doctor; let her/him know you are trying to get pregnant. If you are on any medication then it is wise to include your doctor as early as you can so they can manage any potential complications
- ➢ Do some gentle exercise
- ➢ Have fun trying to get pregnant. Don't make it too stressful and don't worry if you don't get pregnant straightaway. It usually takes up to 6 months to get pregnant and can take a lot longer for some couples.

Remember that if you do experience any problems trying to get pregnant then you can always turn to your doctor, who will be able to offer guidance and help you investigate the cause of any delay.

Now that the sage advice is out of the way, time for me to confess how I got pregnant, and I have to admit that none of my pregnancies were particularly planned. My first pregnancy was a massive shock as I'd been on the pill. I fully admit to being rubbish at taking it consistently though, and would often forget to take it in the morning, then remember as I went to bed that night, or just plain skip a day. Hint to self: if you're taking the pill to stop yourself from getting pregnant then it's a pretty good idea to actually take the darn thing!

Pregnancies 2 and 3 were slightly better planned. We came off the pill and just played a wait and see game, but with both we didn't have to wait long at all. Now some people may read that and think, wow, isn't she lucky. I think the lucky ones are the ones who have partners who are willing to try anything to help the woman achieve her dream, I think the lucky ones are those women whose partners adore their every flaw and I think just because I was able to get pregnant quickly means nothing except I got pregnant quickly. Some women will, and some women won't. Don't beat yourself up if you are struggling to get pregnant. It will happen hopefully, and if you are struggling right now then as I write this I am crossing all my fingers and toes for you and hoping that your dreams come true.

3 THE FIRST TRIMESTER

The First Signs

Are you or aren't you? Some people get a feeling almost immediately that something has happened, some (like me) don't realise until they are well into the first trimester. Some, maybe also like me, ignore the signs and try to convince themselves that it's just something they've eaten – yeah, like you've eaten something 2 weeks ago and you're still feeling funny!? Here are the tell-tale signs:

The earliest and most obvious sign of pregnancy is a missed period, or an abnormally light period. As soon as you think you are late you should take a test to check whether you are pregnant or not.

My periods continued, in a fashion. A tiny bit of blood was enough to allow me to wallow in denial. That and pure ridiculousness. Now I know most women will scoff at what I'm about to admit, but I am rubbish with dates. I don't remember how long has passed between periods – pathetic I know! My brain refuses to work sensibly a lot of the time! Sure, I could keep a note in a journal or diary, but really, I've tried, and I usually then just forget to write in that too. If you are as pathetic as I've just admitted to being, then you need to check out the other symptoms, as it was the nauseous thing that made me realise each and every time.

As well as feeling nauseous, other common symptoms include being physically sick and feeling unusually tired. You may also feel a tingly sensation in your breasts, or increased tenderness.

Compared to a lot of women, I didn't fare too badly. With my first child I completely went off food, particularly in the daytime. I'd find myself having fruit smoothies for lunch with more fruit for dessert.

The weirdest thing I experienced was with regard to a shop. Before I was pregnant I used to go to a particular shop for lunch every day but when I got pregnant I couldn't even walk past the shop without feeling nauseous. I noticed a really strong smell (that nobody else noticed) which turned my stomach. I wasn't very happy about that one as I had to pass the shop at least 3 times every day!

The other symptom that really floored me was the tiredness. My husband noticed it more with the 2nd and 3rd child, he always complained that I would go up to put the first one to sleep and never reappear. That's because I'd end up falling asleep! I was tired throughout the first trimester in each of my pregnancies, and the third trimester, but more of that later.

The tiredness wasn't such an issue with my first pregnancy as it was with the other two as I could easily go home and relax, and I had my fair share of lie-ins. If this is your first pregnancy then I would definitely advise making the most of the odd lie-in, as they will soon become a thing of the past.

In my third pregnancy, I would take the kids up to bed at 7:30 and half the time would not come down again, or my husband would come up to wake me and ask if I was okay. I just felt so exhausted all the time, and regularly felt nauseous, although thankfully I was never actually sick.

One symptom they don't tell you so much, but I definitely experienced, was mood swings. Probably due to the fact that I was so tired, but I was a moody cow! The slightest thing would irritate me; especially anything annoying my husband said or did. The number of fights we had in the first trimesters of our 2 younger children were far too many to remember! The old adage of "don't have a baby to fix your relationship" is absolutely true, if anything, if your relationship isn't strong in the first place the likelihood of a baby strengthening it is simply fanciful.

From the experience of friends and colleagues, I think the worst symptom to suffer from in the early days is vomiting. Thankfully, I didn't suffer with that with any of my pregnancies but I know women who ended up coming into work late most days as they had spent the first hour of the day with their heads in a bowl. If that sounds like you then I hope you get through the first trimester really quick!

Another thing they fail to tell you is that the phrase "morning sickness" is just that: a phrase. "Morning sickness" can happen at any point in the day. My mum used to suffer horrendous morning sickness in the evenings, and a close friend used to wake up feeling fine, but by lunchtime be running to the toilet every 5 minutes.

The vast number of symptoms and general lethargy felt in the first trimester can all be attributed to the fact that you are in the first throes of creating a brand new life. Of course it's going to affect you in some way, and of course you are not going to sail through this massive change in your body without noticing certain changes and experiencing certain feelings and aches and pains. Remembering that each pregnancy is different and each person handles pregnancy in different ways can help a great deal when you're confronted with a perfect pregnancy whilst yours is anything but.

It used to drive me insane when people would assume that because they had gone through something that I must have gone through the same. And there is nothing worse than being compared to a woman who has had an easy pregnancy – there are such things – especially when you are struggling with 101 competing symptoms.

If you do seem to be suffering more than others it can seem like people are judging you for playing on your pregnancy. Don't let the opinions of others make you stressed or upset. I know it's hard to do, but just try to focus on yourself, what you need and ultimately what the baby needs.

When Should You Tell People?

That is a question many people ask and the best answer is: when you are ready. You might be over the moon and bursting to tell the world, and if you are, who's stopping you? You might want to keep it a secret until the 12 week scan in case anything goes wrong, which is more than understandable if you have suffered a previous miscarriage or traumatic pregnancy.

You may be bursting to tell but have been sworn to secrecy by your partner who isn't ready to let the world in on your secret. Every experience is different; you'll know when it feels right to share, and then you can shout it from the rooftops – if you have the energy to climb up there of course!

Did You Know?

Did you know that just 12 weeks after conception your baby is fully formed, with all its organs, bones, limbs, muscles and sex organs being well developed?

Who Should You Tell First?

The obvious answer here is your partner, parents, then siblings and close friends, but you usually tell your best friend first, who may be the one who goes to the chemist with you to buy your first, or tenth, pregnancy kit. You may end up blurting it out to a stranger or someone at work, and your partner may find themselves being way down the list if you have friendships that have lasted a lifetime. Tell who you want first. There is no protocol, or if there is, I certainly don't know of it.

My husband was the first to know on each occasion, purely because I can't keep secrets and I saw him every single day – we lived with each other. My best friend told me she was 4 weeks pregnant, at a time when I was 10 weeks pregnant with our second child and no-one but the hubby and I knew. Why did I keep it from her when she had shared her news with me? Because I wasn't ready to share. Our first pregnancy was a miscarriage that happened at 10 weeks so until the 12 week scan showed everything was okay we told nobody, and we did that with each pregnancy. The thought of telling people and then having to share the bad news as well was enough to convince me that I could keep my secret for a little while longer.

That my boss knew I'd had a miscarriage but my family didn't – I had to explain why I was off work and why it was necessary for me to work from home for a couple of days after – may be a sad indication of the closeness of our family but again, every person and every family is different. If we were all the same the world would certainly be a boring place to live, wouldn't it?

As my first trimesters weren't too horrific I found it quite easy to keep my secret. With my first child I told one friend at work who I usually went out for lunch with, just to explain away the fact that I could no longer eat sandwiches and had to avoid certain places. With my second and third I simply waited until my scan. As soon as I had that picture in my hand I told everyone who would listen.

But what if you are suffering from severe morning sickness or your tiredness is affecting how well you do your job? What do you do then? I would hope that you have an understanding and sympathetic boss and explain your situation, emphasising the fact that you aren't sharing your news yet. If you need to tell your boss early then they should respect your privacy and keep the information to themselves, whilst making provisions for your condition.

Travel

It might seem like a silly thing, particularly if your daily commute involves jumping in your car and driving to work and back, but if you travel on public transport in rush hour, the first trimester can be hell. You're tired, you ache, your energy levels are pathetically low and you really don't want to be standing on a train, bus or the tube for any amount of time. This isn't such a problem once you start to show, or shouldn't be, but in that early stage you look absolutely normal.

Find out if your travel company have special badges or schemes. I travelled into London every day and used the tube, which has a funky little badge you can wear letting people know you're pregnant. The hope is that people will notice your polite little badge and give up their seat for you. You'll be surprised who does and doesn't relinquish their seats.

Rant time: I would expect women to be great at giving up seats, followed by an older generation of men who have had children so remember how uncomfortable their wives/girlfriends were in that stage, but no. The age group I found to be the most polite and helpful were young people, particularly young men. I even had one guy who was standing in a packed tube train with me, ask another man to give up his seat.

I was standing, obviously pregnant at this point, in the middle of the carriage, with everyone's noses down into their books, unwilling to look up and acknowledge that someone else may need the seat just a tiny bit more than they did. My knight in shining armour was a rough looking teenager who obviously had more class than the bankers and city workers who just wanted to exist in their own little cocoons.

Another memorable trip was a train ride back from London. If you've ever ridden a packed train after work then you know exactly what I mean. I stood for 40 minutes, again with a noticeable bump (I must have been about 4.5 months pregnant for this story) until a girl stood up to get off. As she passed she said "I didn't know whether you were pregnant or not so didn't give up my seat in case I offended you". Huh??? So why even mention it now!? That one annoyed me slightly more than others.

I got used to the rudeness of others on my commutes to and from work but for all those out there who are battling through this lack of common courtesy I have two words: reserved seats. I discovered that each carriage has at least 2-4 seats that are marked for passengers with limited movement. This includes the elderly, infirm, those carrying small children, and pregnant women. I took great pleasure in kicking people out of these seats if I walked through a carriage and no-one offered a seat. Don't suffer in silence, it won't hurt anyone to stand up for a while, if you have a legitimate reason for a seat then you have a right to ask for it!

So who were the worst offenders in trying to keep their seats? Easily without a shadow of a doubt it was the middle aged suited and booted 40-50 year old man. I've never seen so many men hide their faces in their books or newspapers, afraid to be asked to give up their precious seat. And I've never before experienced such self-serving idiots.

You will no doubt have your own battles, or develop your own pet peeve about being pregnant. As you can probably tell, mine was travelling. I still get incensed about it now. And as such, I beseech anyone reading this book, if you see a woman who is pregnant, whether it is wearing a badge or wearing a prominent bump, please offer her your seat, or whatever other help she may need. I guarantee it will be greatly appreciated.

First Trimester Pregnancy Symptoms

Some of these have been further up in the first trimester section but I thought it was worth running through them again in a much more official sounding way to make sure I get the main facts across. Of course if you are worried about any of these symptoms, or anything else for that matter, the best thing you can do is book an appointment with your doctor or midwife and discuss your concerns with them. As an additional point of reference there are many fantastic websites out there that cover pregnancy, just type "pregnancy" into your search engine of choice and you'll have a list longer than your arm.

Constipation
Due to hormonal changes you can get constipated in the early stages of pregnancy. If you do, try eating foods high in fibre such as brown bread, wholemeal pasta and rice, wholegrain cereals and fruit and vegetables. Drink plenty of water and if you are still suffering try limiting the amount of iron you consume – though you may need to check this with your doctor if you are on iron supplements.

Feeling faint
Again due to those pesky hormonal changes, you may feel faint. Try not

to stand still for too long or get up too quickly from a chair or out of a hot bath. You can also feel faint when lying on your back and if you do try simply turning onto your side. Don't lie on your back in the later stages of pregnancy; it's not good for your baby.

Itching
Due to the increased blood supply to the skin you may find yourself a lot itchier than usual, and even a lot hotter. Wearing loose clothes will help particularly natural fibres.

Nose bleeds
Nose bleeds are a common occurrence during pregnancy due to hormonal changes and usually don't last long. As long as you don't lose a lot of blood there is nothing to worry about.

Passing urine
Needing to go to the toilet more often usually starts during early pregnancy and continues right through until the birth. As your pregnancy develops the urge to pee is due to your baby's head pressing on your bladder. Whilst on the toilet if you rock in a back and forth motion you will lessen the pressure of your uterus on your bladder meaning you can empty it properly.

Piles
One of the lovelier effects of pregnancy is itchy little lumps known as piles or haemorrhoids. They are caused by your veins relaxing as your hormones kick in and can make going to the toilet uncomfortable, even sometimes resulting in a little blood. They usually go after labour but to relieve any discomfit you should avoid standing for long periods of time, exercise regularly and eat foods high in fibre. Drinking lots of water will also help as piles are linked to constipation. Apparently if you feel a pile then you should gently push it back inside with some lubricating jelly.

I am so glad that this isn't one of the symptoms I experienced, and hope anyone who is experiencing it gets over it quick as it sounds horrible!

Skin and hair changes
The first thing you'll probably notice in this department is that your nipples will darken, and may even appear bigger. Your hair also grows more and I was fortunate enough to be one of those who developed a noticeable line of hair from my abdomen down to you know where. Nice! Never have wax strips come in more useful. I also discovered an errant chin hair would

pop up every few weeks, in the exact same place. I didn't expect to be growing chin hair until I was in my late 60s so thanks for that one Mother Nature.

Everything does settle down and go back to normal once the baby arrives but in the meantime, keep an eye on the usual stuff – moles, freckles, lumps and bumps – and make sure you use extra sun cream as you may also find that you tan more easily.

Talking about hair growth, one side effect of pregnancy that I didn't know about is that you grow more hair on the top of your head too, so chances are that you will catch a few compliments on how lovely and thick it's looking. What I didn't realise is that that hair will also come out…in clumps! I remember after my first child washing my hair in the shower and finding a huge mass of hair coming away as I was getting the suds out. I freaked out – who wouldn't! The same freaking out I did when I found my first grey pubic hair! I had a grey pubic hair before I even had a grey hair on my head. And yes, "had" is definitely the right tense to use as on spotting it I swiftly tweezered it away as if it had never happened. Only you and I know about that one.

Teeth

I hear you now asking, is it every part of my body that will get affected by this pregnancy? The short answer: yes. And that includes your teeth, and more specifically, your gums.

We've all seen the dental floss and toothpaste ads showing us the build-up of plaque on our teeth which leads to bleeding gums. Your hormones can cause that plaque to make your gums more inflamed. Bleeding gums are quite common so make sure you are extra vigilant when brushing and flossing and try to avoid any sugary drinks or food.

Vaginal discharge

It's nothing new and most of us will experience it. It shouldn't smell too nasty and should be clear and white but if this isn't the case you may have an infection such as thrush. Let your doctor or midwife know, trust me, they'll be used to hearing about it and will be able to help you treat it quickly and simply.

Bleeding

Bleeding during pregnancy can come at any stage. Bleeding in the first few months can be a sign of an ectopic pregnancy or miscarriage – this was the first thing that alerted me that something may be wrong. When I got pregnant again I had another bleeding scare and convinced myself that the unthinkable had happened again, but no, it was just as a result of a little bit of hanky panky.

If you do have an early scare you will probably be offered an early scan. These can be a bit scary as if it is really early in your pregnancy sometimes the heartbeat of your baby can't be seen. This doesn't mean that there is no heartbeat just that your baby is so small that sometimes it simply can't be detected yet.

With my miscarriage, I had a viability scan (early scan) at about 7 weeks and was told I would have to come back 2 weeks later as they couldn't detect anything. Those 2 weeks were the longest 2 weeks of my life, waiting and wondering and hoping. When I saw the look on the technician's face I knew it was bad news and I was quickly booked in for a D&C a week later.

On coming out of the hospital after being told that news I found a parking ticket on my car, which had been given because I was 10 minutes late back to the car. You can imagine how upset that made me!

Anyway, a D&C, or dilatation and curettage to give it its proper name, is a minor surgical procedure that removes the tissue and anything else from the lining of your womb. I was offered one because I was going on holiday only a few weeks later and was advised to have one to make sure the miscarriage completed. So not only did I have the incredible pain of expelling my baby and the massive amounts of blood that came with it, I also had to endure a surgical procedure. That was not a good month for me!

If you have also experienced a miscarriage, or are worried about whether you may miscarry, you are not alone. It must be the number one worry amongst pregnant women everywhere, and statistics declare that 1 in 4 first pregnancies will miscarry.

It sounds like there is a lot NOT to look forward to, but for most women the first trimester passes by pretty quickly. Women don't tend to find out they are pregnant until about week 6 so you are already half way through the first trimester.

You won't get every symptom; you may not even get three. You're pretty much bound to get stuck with at least one of these symptoms though. If the symptoms bother you enough to warrant a doctor's visit then don't be embarrassed just ask for help and they will likely find a way to try and alleviate your problem.

The second trimester is just around the corner and before you know it you'll be feeling better than ever.

What to Eat and What to Avoid

There is a lot of information about what foods to eat, and what ones to avoid, but it should go without saying that upping your intake of fruits and vegetables can only be a good thing. Try and stick to the food wheel guidelines – you want to be eating about 30% fruit and vegetables, 30% meat and proteins, 30% bread, rice, and pasta and 10% naughty stuff. And don't kid yourself, naughty stuff includes chocolate, biscuits and cake!

In my first pregnancy I was advised to stay clear of nuts but by the time I was pregnant with my third child that advice was no longer given. It strikes me as bloody ironic that I craved peanuts in my first pregnancy, but wasn't bothered by them at all in my second and third pregnancies.

So what food should you avoid? Unfortunately, there's quite a lot of it, and some of it is my favourite stuff! Like soft cheese: I love cheese smothered onto crusty bread and French stick. My favourite is that spreadable blue cheese, which is a big no-no apparently.

Of course, once you've had your baby you can eat as much of it as you want! I was even told to pig out on cheese, milk products and chocolate (especially hot chocolate) to encourage my milk to come in. Not sure how scientific that one is, but it made me feel good to eat and drink lots of comforting foods, and surely fatty foods can help encourage your milk? No? Well I'm choosing to believe that a little of a bad thing can be very good indeed – all in moderation of course!

It will come as no surprise that all pregnant, and breastfeeding, women are advised to avoid alcohol and drugs. Now I'm not going to lie and say I never drank an alcoholic drink throughout my pregnancies and whilst breastfeeding, but I never had more than one drink, and I never drank consistently. I had the odd one to celebrate an anniversary or party, and a little half glass of wine with meals sometimes, but that was it. I think if you can moderate yourself and not, NEVER, EVER, have more than one, then you will be fine with the odd drink. However, if you can't stop after one then just don't have any. It's not worth it. Why risk your child's health for the sake of a couple of drinks? It's like drink driving – it's just NOT WORTH IT!!!

Apologies for the lecture but I don't think many people will disagree, and whilst I didn't want to pretend I was a total teetotaller, I also want to make clear that I don't condone drinking regularly whilst being pregnant, or having young children.

Lecture over with, let's get down to the dos and don'ts:

DO EAT FRUIT AND VEGETABLES: All health agencies will advise you to eat at least 5 portions of fruit and vegetables per day, and these can be fresh, canned, frozen or in a juice. If you want to make sure you get the maximum nutrients out of your fruit and vegetables then it is advised that you eat them raw or lightly cooked. Easy enough for fruit, but if you're wondering what to do about your veggies then apparently steaming them is best.

DO EAT CARBOHYDRATES: Carbohydrates such as bread, potatoes, rice, and pasta, are another source of vitamins and fibre and should make up the main part of your meal. To be ultra-healthy with your carbs try eating the wholegrain varieties. We swapped out our penne and fusilli pasta for the wholegrain variety, and even the kids don't notice the difference.

DO EAT MILK AND DAIRY: Milk, yoghurt and cheese contain calcium and other nutrients needed by your baby. Word of caution though, check out the DO NOTS as there are some types of cheese (soft cheese particularly) that you are not supposed to eat. Cheeses that you can eat include hard cheeses such as cheddar and parmesan, and processed cheese such as mozzarella, cheese spread and cottage cheese. If in doubt, seek advice or just don't eat it.

DO EAT FISH, EGGS, MEAT AND BEANS: This food source is vital for protein and other sources of nutrients. While this food source shouldn't constitute the bulk of your daily diet it is advisable that you eat moderate amounts every day. It is massively important to make sure that all your food is thoroughly cooked as you don't want to be suffering from food poisoning during your pregnancy. Try to eat 2 portions of fish per week, and try to make one of those portions of the oily kind. Oily fish you can eat include fresh tuna, mackerel, salmon, trout and sardines.

On the food wheel the other food type is food and drink high in fat and sugar. By that, I always read "the naughty stuff I can't live without". Think chocolate, crisps, biscuits, ice cream, salad dressings and oils, you know, all the stuff you crave even when not pregnant!

Obviously these high-fat and high-sugar foods are not good for us, and we should not be eating a lot of them, but in moderation they are okay. By moderation I don't mean a 4 pack of chocolate eclairs (yes, I have!) nor do I mean a whole pack of biscuits (yet to accomplish that feat!), but 1 or 2.

Eating more sugary or fatty foods will lead to weight gain, and don't kid yourself about the whole "eating for 2" thing, it's not an excuse, and you WILL find it harder to shift the pregnancy weight once baby is here.

If anything, we should all try to cut down on this food type, remembering that the onset of diabetes in pregnancy is rising, and the more fatty foods we consume the higher the amount of bad cholesterol in our blood, increasing our chances of developing heart disease.

Okay, so now the foods to avoid, and notice I put the sugary/fatty stuff in the DOs and not the DON'Ts? We can eat these foods, heck I couldn't survive a day without some kind of naughty treat.

Women are advised not to eat the foods listed below because of their potential to harm your baby or make you ill. Don't be scared, this is precautionary it is better to prevent illness rather than have to treat it.

DON'T EAT TYPES OF CHEESE: Avoid soft cheese such as Brie, Camembert and soft blue cheese. The reason why is because they are made with mould and can contain listeria which is a type of bacteria that could harm your baby.

DON'T EAT PATE: For the same reasons as soft cheese – it can contain listeria.

DON'T EAT RAW OR PARTLY COOKED EGGS: Eggs must be cooked through to prevent the risk of salmonella food poisoning. This includes avoiding home-made mayonnaise.

DON'T EAT RAW OR UNDERCOOKED MEAT: Make sure there is no trace of pink or blood in your meat, and that any meat juices run clear. This particularly applies to minced meat and sausages, though eating steaks and other whole cuts of beef or lamb can be eaten rare so long as they are properly cooked or sealed.

DON'T EAT LIVER: Now this was one I hadn't come across before and I don't remember ever avoiding liver during any of my pregnancies, but apparently eating liver or liver pâté can be harmful to your baby due to the amount of vitamin A it contains.

DON'T EAT SOME TYPES OF FISH: You shouldn't eat shark, marlin, swordfish or more than 2 tuna steaks per week (or more than 4 cans of tuna per week). The reason is due to the high levels of mercury in these fish which can damage the developing nervous system of your baby. This is also why it is advised to eat only 2 portions of oily fish per week.

DON'T EAT RAW SHELLFISH: They can contain harmful bacteria and viruses that cause food poisoning.

DON'T DRINK UNPASTEURISED MILK: The advice is that you should only drink pasteurised or UHT milk, and if you do have to drink any other kind of milk you should boil it first. You are also advised not to eat any foods made from unpasteurised milk, such as soft goats' cheese.

When I was pregnant with my first child I was warned not to eat peanuts. I'm not sure what the reasoning behind it is but you are now told that you can eat peanuts, in moderation. I heard from someone that the reason why they stopped recommending no peanuts was because they found lots of newborn were developing allergies to peanuts as they hadn't been exposed to them whilst inside the womb. Now I don't know whether that is true or whether it's just a silly story but to my uneducated mind it kind of makes sense. Scientifically speaking, according to the latest research, there is no direct link between eating or not eating peanuts and your baby developing a peanut allergy, and this is why the advice was changed to allow peanuts.

DON'T TAKE SUPPLEMENTS CONTAINING VITAMIN A: Too much vitamin A can harm your baby so make sure to stay away from any supplements containing this vitamin. If you stick to multivitamin supplements specifically created for pregnant ladies then you should be fine, otherwise check the label.

If you're wondering what vitamins you can or should take then the list is below:

Folic acid is one of the most important supplements you can take during pregnancy as it reduces the risk of neural tube defects such as spina bifida. You should start taking folic acid as soon as you start trying for a baby and not stop until you are 12 weeks pregnant. As well as taking the supplement you should also try adding folic acid to your diet by eating more green leafy vegetables, like broccoli and spinach, and brown rice. In certain cases you will need to take bigger doses of folic acid, and if you have specific concerns ask your local doctor.

Vitamin D is also essential during pregnancy as it helps strengthen bones and keep teeth healthy. Without vitamin D your child's bones can soften and they can develop rickets. Whilst there are only a few foods that contain vitamin D, such as fortified breakfast cereals and oily fish, the best source of vitamin D is direct sunlight. Don't think this is a green light to spend the next few weeks sunbathing, though if you live in the UK that won't be a problem as we very rarely have 2 consecutive days of sunshine, let alone weeks of it! Whilst the amount of time you need to spend in the sun to consume your recommended amount of vitamin D varies from person to person, it is less time than it would take to cause any tanning or burning.

Iron deficiency is extremely common during pregnancy and as a result most pregnancy multivitamin supplements will include iron, but even so you may need more. If you find yourself tireder than usual then go and get yourself checked out at the doctors as you may have developed an iron deficiency or have become anaemic.

You may be prescribed additional iron supplements. If you want to add iron to your diet through food you can add green, leafy vegetables to your diet, along with lean meat and dried fruit and nuts. A lot of breakfast cereals also have iron included in them.

Vitamin C helps us absorb iron so add citrus fruits, broccoli, potatoes, blackcurrants, tomatoes and peppers to your diet as all these foods contain vitamin C. Drinking fresh fruit juices will also help if you have low iron levels.

Calcium is needed for making your baby's bones and teeth. Eat dried fruits, bread, cereals, almonds, tofu and green leafy vegetables to up your calcium intake. Oily fish like sardines also contain calcium.

Did you notice a recurring pattern through the foods you should be eating and the vitamins and minerals you should be consuming? I think the message is, eat enough fruit and vegetables, lean, well-cooked meats, oily fish and good carbohydrates and you'll be giving your baby an optimal environment in which to grow.

If you're after ideas for healthy snacks to try to reduce your naughty food intake then try adding some fresh fruit, salad vegetables like carrots or cucumbers, yoghurt, or dried fruits to your diet.

For some quick lunch ideas how about some hummus and pitta bread, or taramasalata and crusty bread, salads, soups, or ham/cheese/tuna sandwiches. For a quick and healthy lunch idea try sardines on toast or baked beans on toast or a baked potato. An omelet filled with veggies is also a good idea, but remember, the eggs need to be thoroughly cooked.

For dinner ideas, try salmon or tuna steaks one night with boiled potatoes and curly kale or broccoli. Pork fillet is delicious, easy to cook and lean. Make homemade burgers, ensuring that you thoroughly cook the meat, and add salad and tomato to your bun. Try your hand at a kedgeree dish or cook up a delicious Sunday roast. We end up having chicken at least 4 nights out of 7 in our house, and if I can't think of anything else to have, I always end up making chicken. It easy, it's quick, and it's one of the healthiest meats you can eat.

For drinks, try unsweetened fruit juice or milky drinks.

So how about our favourite start-to-the-day drinks? You can still drink tea and coffee, you just might not be advised to drink as much as you're used to. Did you know that high levels of caffeine can lead to low birth weights and increased risks of health problems in later life. Too much caffeine can even cause miscarriage so take it seriously when your doctor says you need to cut down on your tea drinking. The advice is to limit your caffeine intake to 2 cups of coffee or 3 cups of tea per day, but remember that caffeine is also found in chocolate and some soft drinks and energy drinks so you can't substitute tea with a coke! The official limit is 200mg of caffeine per day so if you have one bar of plain chocolate and a cup of filter coffee you'd have reached your limit already!

I found this one of the hardest things to do as I'm a heavy tea drinker. I usually have 3 or 4 before lunch and usually another 3 in the evening, and that's not even counting the afternoon! Yep, I'm a caffeine addict, as well as a chocoholic, so you can imagine how much caffeine is pumping round my system!

We started drinking decaffeinated tea after 4pm, which helped, and I tried drinking more water instead of tea. Not the same at all though! If you pick well the decaffeinated tastes exactly the same as the caffeinated. If you try it and it tastes disgusting you've just picked the wrong one, try a few as there will be one that is just as good. Personally I think PG Tips and the own brand supermarket ones are pretty good.

What else should you try and stop?

It goes without saying that if you smoke, stop! I've known pregnant women who carried on smoking, and they have loads of good excuses for continuing to do so. One even told me that their midwife said that they could continue if they didn't inhale properly. Really? Why would you endanger your baby just so you can continue dragging on a poison stick?

Okay, so I don't smoke. I never have. I dabbled a bit when I was younger, and thought I looked cool on a Saturday night with a fag in one hand and a drink in the other, but I never really inhaled properly and thankfully it went no further than that.

My hubby on the other hand does smoke, though not all the time. He smokes when he's having a beer, so maybe 2 or 3 nights a week. But it drives me crazy. He's been trying to stop ever since I've known him, but he still continues to smoke if he's drinking. I'm not about to weigh down on addiction, as apart from caffeine and chocolate I've never been addicted to anything in my life. And I do understand that it is really difficult to quit smoking, I watched both my parents take about 10 years to finally give up smoking, going from one thing to the next trying to kick the habit. And I'm watching the same thing now with the hubby, going from cigars to roll ups to the new-fangled electric cigarette, but he's still buying those Marlboro Lights!

I hate it. He comes in from the garden after a cigarette and then wants to know why I go crazy when he then picks the baby up for a cuddle. Did you know that cigarette smoke can linger on your clothes for over an hour, and what is your baby going to do when being held, yep, snuggle in for a cuddle?

So if you're still smoking and don't really want to give up, let me see if I can shock you with some little known facts:

> - Did you know that you will experience less morning sickness if you stop smoking?
> - Did you know you will experience fewer complications during your pregnancy if you stop smoking?
> - Did you know you will cope better with the birth if you stop smoking?
> - Did you know you are more likely to have a healthier pregnancy and baby if you stop smoking?
> - Did you know you will reduce the risk of still birth if you stop smoking?
> - Did you know that your baby will cope better with any birth complications if you stop smoking?
> - Did you know that it is less likely that your baby will be born prematurely if you stop smoking?
> - Did you know your baby is less likely to be born underweight if

you stop smoking?

➢ Did you know that on average, babies of mothers who smoke are about 8oz or 200g lighter than other babies, and these babies may have problems during and after labour and are also more prone to infection?

➢ Did you known that premature babies often have to deal with breathing difficulties, feeding difficulties and health problems?

➢ Did you know you will reduce the risk of cot death if you stop smoking?

➢ Did you know that children who have parents who smoke are more likely to suffer from illnesses which need hospital treatment, such as asthma?

➢ The sooner you stop the better, but did you know that even if you stop in the last weeks of your pregnancy you will still be benefitting your baby, and yourself?

➢ Did you know second-hand smoke, from your partner, can also affect you and the baby, and can also lead to low birth weight and cot death?

A scary statistic for one final guilt trip: Did you know that children are more likely to be admitted to hospital for pneumonia and bronchitis during their first year of life if their parents smoke, and that over 17,000 children under the age of 5 are admitted to hospital every year due to the effects of second-hand smoke?

And yes, I have shown these statistics to the hubby, who quite frankly, should be ashamed of himself! Addiction is most definitely one of the hardest things to overcome!

So what about that other massively addictive and utterly legal substance – alcohol? Well, no surprises those health agencies also advise against drinking alcohol whilst pregnant and breastfeeding. Did you know that when you drink alcohol it reaches your baby via the placenta and too much of it can seriously affect your baby's development. You only have to think about how awful you feel the next day after a night of drinking to know that it can't be good for a baby who is trying to grow inside your womb.

If possible, avoid alcohol altogether. Now I admit to ignoring the advice to avoid alcohol altogether and instead sit comfortably in the "if you need to drink limit your drinking to 1 to 2 units of alcohol once or twice a week" camp. No, I don't "need" to drink, but I think if you are sensible then there is little wrong with having a glass of wine once or twice a week. Some people will be as incensed with me at that as I am with people who smoke, and yes, maybe I'm a hypocrite, but I, rightly or wrongly, am sticking by the "red wine is good for you if drunk in moderation" party line.

A scary fact though is that your baby's liver is one of the last organs to develop, and doesn't do so until the later stages of pregnancy, meaning that your baby is unable to process alcohol as well as you and I can. The stark reality of this fact alone has made me think maybe my above defence is completely wrong so I'm in no fit state to pass judgement on anyone!

Whilst drinking little and infrequently may be deemed acceptable, drinking heavily throughout your pregnancy can lead to a condition known as Fetal Alcohol Syndrome (FAS), which has such devastating side effects as restricted growth, facial abnormalities and learning and behavioural disorders. Drinking more than 1 or 2 units a week or binge drinking can lead to less severe forms of FAS. You have been warned!

Don't give in to peer pressure, don't let 1 or 2 become 3 or 4 and don't believe that if you do it just a handful of times it won't make a difference. It does, so don't! And yes, I have shouted at myself too!

Another obvious big no no is drugs. Whilst most people realise that cocaine and heroin are not going to be safe for your baby, some may be under the illusion that cannabis will be. It won't. It's illegal for a reason.

I don't really know enough about drugs to make any informed judgement on them – I've led a rather sheltered life – but if you have any questions or concerns speak to your doctor. If they can't help they will be able to point you towards someone who can.

If you take any prescribed or over the counter medication you should also speak to your doctor to make sure they are safe for your baby. Make sure any health professional you are dealing with knows you are pregnant, and this includes dentists and even alternative health therapists like herbalists and masseurs!

Exercising

One of the questions you will be asked when you go for your regular pre-natal appointments is "what exercises are you doing?" I've never really been an exercise person. I hate running and honestly feel like I could pass out if I even run round the block. That said I can do 30 minutes on a cross trainer and not be puffed even half as much as if I'd ran for 2 minutes. Some people surely must be more suited to one type of exercise than another, and I most definitely will never be running a marathon, or even a 5k race!

I've tried gyms. I hate them. I hate having to think about what I'm going to wear and how I'm going to look, and how to work the machines without looking like an idiot.

I can't swim, so that form of exercise is out, although that is apparently an excellent exercise to do if you are pregnant. I think I'm also the only woman who hates swimming purely because it means I've got to make sure I'm presentable before going – errant hairs not being classified as a good look these days.

I have 3 preschoolers to look after and run around after now, and I happen to think that is more exercise than I'll ever need. Add to that the fact that I have to clean the house and the mess the kids make every day and I think I'm doing pretty well.

I want to pretend and say I walk a lot but the truth is; I don't. When my eldest started school I had all these grand plans about walking to school – a 25 minute walk – but I think I've walked about 10 times in the whole school year, which is now close to finishing.

Exercise is important, especially when you're pregnant, as you need to be as fit as you can be. I wish I was fitter, I wish I could run up the 2 flights of stairs in our house without puffing and panting when I got to the top, I wish I was that mum with the hourglass figure who everyone envied, but I'm not. I get my exercise from running around after the kids and keeping the house in order. I reckon that probably constitutes more than the recommended 30 minutes exercise per day, so I can't be doing that badly.

If you are like me then as long as you are not sitting on your bum all day I think we'll live. Maintain a healthy weight and try and do some type of activity at the weekend and make sure your kids get some exercise and eat a balanced diet and you'll be doing better than most.

If you do want to do more, then I commend you. If you want to try something light then consider something like pregnancy yoga or Pilates, or a prenatal swim exercise class. I did pregnancy yoga when pregnant with my first child, and I really enjoyed it. Once my second was on his way, I found it hard to get away.

The problem is that when you have kids, dedicating yourself to a time-sensitive weekly activity is hard, especially when you don't have a solid support network. The hubby isn't always home at a time when I would want to do exercise classes, you can't do them with the kids in tow, and by the time you've got them in bed you're often too tired to even think about exercising, let alone doing anything about it.

Okay, I may be making excuses for myself, I know that. But I carried on doing yoga at home when I found myself with a few extra minutes. I even tried doing the New York City ballet DVD, which I really enjoyed. I'm not one for the more active exercise DVDs, I worry I'm going to look stupid if the hubby walked in.

If I found myself thinking about it throughout the day I would do some pelvic floor exercises. Now they are just plain easy, and I would definitely recommend doing some of those, especially if you want to control any leaking of the pee variety!

The pelvic floor is placed under great strain during pregnancy and childbirth and can weaken considerably, and this is what causes a little pee to escape when you cough or sneeze. If you strengthen it with these little tips then you will normally experience less escaping pee.

How do you do a pelvic exercise? My midwife told me to simply clench your pee muscle 10 times in quick succession. Not know which muscle that is? Next time you pee try to stop mid-flow. That is your pelvic floor muscle, and that movement you did to stop your pee is a pelvic exercise.

If you want to be a bit more serious about it then stand with your shoulders and bum against a wall. Bend your knees slightly and pull your belly button towards your spine so your back is flat against the wall. Hold for 5 seconds and release. Repeat 10 times.

Try to do pelvic exercises at least 3 times a day. It doesn't matter where, you can even do it sitting on the bus and no-one would ever know.

If you are suffering from this condition, which is officially known as stress incontinence, then ask your midwife or doctor about it.

Strengthening your abdominal muscles is also a recommended exercise as it can help to ease backache, an extremely common complaint during pregnancy.

As your baby grows you will find your back muscles coming under more and more stress and so anything you can do to ease your discomfit can only be good.

Get down on all fours (pretend you are a cat!), with your hands under your shoulders and your knees under your hips. Your fingers should be pointing forward and your stomach muscles should be tight so your back is straight.

From the straight back position, breathe out pushing your back into a slight arch and let your head fall down. It should be a gentle movement. Breathe in and bring your head back and straighten your back so you have a straight line from the top of your head to the base of your spine.

Hold each pose for a few seconds and work the movements with your breathe; steady and slow. Repeat 10 times. If you do yoga you may recognise this as a light version of the cat pose. You should never feel out of breathe or uncomfortable doing this movement.

Another simple exercise that can help another common complaint is to do with the feet. Exercising your feet can improve blood circulation, prevent cramp in your calf muscles and reduce swelling in your ankles.

Leg cramps appear to be a common side effect of pregnancy, and you may even find yourself woken in the night by agonising cramps. I hated this part of pregnancy as they are really painful, and got worse as my pregnancies progressed.

So how can we relieve the pain? Bend and stretch one foot up then down 30 times. Then rotate your foot round in a clockwise movement 8 times, and then repeat the movement anti-clockwise. Do the exact same movements on your other foot.

Summary

So that's most of the first trimester covered. We've discussed diet, health, exercise, common symptoms, and how to tell if you're pregnant or not.

The end of your first trimester will be marked by the scan and it is after this event that you are likely to start sharing your news, if you haven't done so before.

As you move into your second trimester, you will start to show and may even have to go out shopping for maternity clothes – not always a fun event! Your first trimester symptoms and complaints should now start to slowly melt away and you'll start to feel much better physically. And no, it doesn't last!

4 THE SECOND TRIMESTER

Did You Know?
During the second trimester a woman has 50% more blood than before her pregnancy.

It is by about week 16 that you should start feeling a lot better and the symptoms that plagued your early pregnancy should fade away. People call the second trimester the honeymoon period, due to the fact that the first trimester symptoms dissipate and the uncomfortable waddling of the third trimester has yet to happen.

The best part of the second trimester though is what happens around the 18-20 weeks mark. It is at this stage that you first start feeling your baby kick. From about week 18-20 you will start to feel small fluttering movements. In all honesty, at first you may put the feelings down to wind or indigestion, but you'll soon notice them growing stronger and before long your partner will be able to feel them too.

Your first proper pregnancy (I'm not counting my official first one as that was so short-lived and afforded me none of the pleasures of the second trimester) feels so special and you can't help but feel special yourself, like you stand out in the crowd all of a sudden, and are someone with a purpose and a reason to be.

I loved rubbing my belly, patting my belly, affectionately talking to it and bonding with the baby who was growing inside me. The other fantastic thing about the second trimester is that your other half also starts to notice the changes, and as your belly gets bigger, he starts to get more and more attentive. Every night hubby would use the special cocoa butter stretchmark cream and spend at least 10 minutes rubbing my belly and talking softly to it. He bought a book that he would read each night to it as we'd read that baby can hear things that are going on outside and can recognise Dad's voice.

My advice: Take advantage of this new found specialness. Luxuriate in the feeling of creating something amazing, and take any chance you can to relax and unwind and let people look after you. If your other half tries to do too much let him! By the time the second one comes along he'll think it's nothing unusual and you'll find yourself getting little attention at all.

I remember fondly the days of my first full pregnancy, how attentive the hubby was and how involved he wanted to be with everything, from midwives appointments to applying the cream to my belly and ensuring I was taking my Pregnacare vitamins. When pregnant with my second child the attentiveness waned somewhat and my belly was rubbed every few days rather than every night. He only came to the important midwife/hospital appointments, and the running around after the poor pregnant missus bit was a thing of the past.

By the time of my third full pregnancy, the attentiveness was all but gone. Yes, I was amazing doing all that I was doing, but that was on a good day when he felt like giving compliments. It was status quo, and most days played out exactly the same as if I'd have been the most non-pregnant person in the world. I can count the number of times I have had my belly rubbed this time, and only the hospital scan visits now qualify for partner accompaniment. If I'm tired it's just an annoyance rather than a cute trait of pregnancy. Oh how things change!

So be warned ladies, take advantage of all the extra love. It may not last! And for any men out there reading this, a pregnancy is a pregnancy. We still feel as tired as we did with our first, we still want our feet rubbed and our cream applied, and we still want to feel special and wonderful. Step up!

If I had to choose one favourite time during each of my pregnancies, every time it would be the second trimester. I loved this stage of pregnancy! The horrible nausea of the first trimester went and my energy levels went back to normal. I started feeling like myself again and had told everyone about the impending arrival. It is at this stage that you start to feel really special. Everyone you come into contact with comments on how you look and you can't help but enjoy it. Sure you may get some smug so-and-so mention a weight gain but as soon as you state the reason why they're usually full of congratulatory rhetoric.

Baby Moving

If you are unsure whether the movements you are feeling are the baby moving or not then you can always check with your midwife, but they'll usually tell you that if it feels different then chances are it's your baby.

This is the time when you'll find your hand constantly resting on your stomach. I get all misty-eyed just thinking about how special I used to feel carrying around a brand new human with unknown potential and the chance to be whoever they want to be.

My husband was massively jealous that I was getting to feel the baby move around whilst he could only look on so the next best feeling to the first movements is the look on their faces when your partner gets to feel baby for the first time. At that point you'll be used to the feelings and be full of confidence.

If you are at the early 'is he/she moving or isn't he/she moving' stage then by the time baby can be felt by another you'll know for sure whether they are kicking or not. You'll be the wise old owl showing the new employee how things work.

Chances are your partner will be in awe of this new development and want to stroke and touch your belly as much as you do. While this attention may be welcomed it's the attention you'll get from everyone else that may drive you insane.

Whether this is a new societal development or whether people have been doing this same thing for generations, but once you start to show people tend to treat you like public property, or at least they treat your stomach as such.

Watch out for the little old ladies who try to rub your belly, or the work colleagues who rush over to 'have a go' when you jump from a kick. I've had people – strangers – approach me in shops trying to rub my belly before and asking a myriad of personal questions about how far along you are and whether I'm expecting twins or not.

Which brings me to my next moan… if you look further along than you are, i.e. if your bump is progressing well, then you'll be asked whether you're expecting twins. Why everyone says this is beyond me, but I have to confess just the other day on seeing my neighbour and finding out how far along she was, I committed the same offence and asked "Are you sure it's not twins in there?"

I don't know why I said it, I used to hate it when people said it to me, maybe it's an inbuilt response we all have? There were times when, after responding with the "No, there aren't twins in there, I've had the scan and there's only one" answer, I was told that maybe the twin was hiding behind his/her brother/sister. Really?!? The scans are so detailed now that they can tell you whether your baby may have a potential medical problem or not but they can't tell you whether there's another baby hiding behind the first one? Come on people, isn't it time we stopped using that phrase!?

Did you know?

Your baby will grow faster between weeks 15 and 22 than at any other time in their lives?

Growing Bump

At first when you start showing, it just looks like you've put on weight. As the weeks pass your bump will grow bigger and bigger. You will also start to show around this time; although every woman and every pregnancy is different so don't judge yourself on what is happening to others. Your uterus is expanding to allow for the growth of your baby and your appetite may also start to increase.

Some people put weight on everywhere, others just seem to add to their ever-expanding bellies, and others notice massive changes in their bust area. Wherever you put the weight on, don't worry about it. If you eat healthily and maintain some form of an exercise regime then chances are you will be able to get rid of it once the baby arrives.

TIP: The best way to get rid of baby weight post labour? Breastfeeding!

When you breastfeed the muscles in your uterus contract, speeding along the process of losing the belly weight. Another massive bonus when breastfeeding is that the typical calories it takes to feed in any given day is 500. 500 calories! What better excuse do you need, other than the fact that it is the best possible start your baby could ever wish for?

I really struggled throughout my pregnancy with maintaining a healthy diet as I found myself constantly wanting to eat chocolate, particularly with my third child. In my first pregnancy I craved oranges and drank lots of delicious fruit smoothies, but in my third pregnancy I just wanted to drink chocolate milkshakes and eat chocolate bars. Thankfully I had 2 other children to keep me busy and give me enough exercise to burn off the excess calories, but I hate to think what my arteries look like now!

The hubby did make sure I also ate lots of healthy foods and I did temper the chocolate intake with lots of fruit.

Did you know?

Your baby's face is now becoming much more defined, with their hair, eyebrows and eyelashes now beginning to grow.

Enjoy your second trimester, it's a lovely time. This is the trimester where you get to feel your baby kick for the first time, you'll have regular check-ups with your midwife and get to hear the baby's heartbeat and see your bump growing bigger by the day. Splash out on some maternity outfits and embrace the bump.

My Beating Heart

Hearing your baby's heartbeat is another massive milestone right up there with feeling your baby's kick for the first time. At each and every prenatal appointment, your midwife or doctor will check your blood pressure and perform a quick check on baby by feeling your stomach and listening to their heartbeat. Every single time this happens is like the first time, and each time it takes them a couple of seconds to locate the beat of their heart is the scary moment when you wonder whether everything is alright. It happened to me every time. They put the gel on your stomach and scan for their heartbeat. It usually takes a few seconds so don't be alarmed if you don't hear the beating of their heart within the first second or two.

For the first couple of midwife appointments I'd suggest asking your partner if they want to come along. They don't have to join you for each check-up, but the first time you hear the heartbeat is just one of those times when you want them to be there with you, listening along and sharing that secret smile. The smile that says everything is alright with the world and our baby is coming along just fine.

New Wardrobe

If you don't invite them to every prenatal appointment you probably won't want them tagging along to your shopping excursions to bag yourself some very fetching maternity clothes. Don't treat maternity clothes shopping like any other shopping event. Maternity clothes are usually not the height of fashion, and you will be massively limited in your options.

Unless you have a lot of money to spend you will want to be choosing your options carefully and narrowing your selection down to the absolute necessary. If you are still working through your pregnancy then you are going to need one or two pairs of maternity trousers or skirts. Two or three work tops should be enough, though you could also try buying the next size up in baggy free flowing tops if you'd prefer. With my second pregnancy I was the biggest during the summer months so found maternity shopping quite easy as the loose fitting spaghetti strap tops were all the rage. I managed to kit myself out for next to nothing.

Maternity jeans are another must-have I think, and I wouldn't have been without mine. If you can, get 2 pairs just so you can change them up occasionally, and if it's summer invest in some leggings and open cardigans to complete your look.

I swear by cardigans, particularly if you are going to be breastfeeding. They provide cover for feeding mums and can make it look like your merely holding your baby if you wear them right. I think by this point I'm probably known as the cardigan girl but who cares, they're comfy and practical and at this point that's all I'm worried about.

Blue or Pink?

The biggest decision of your second trimester will be whether you want to know the sex of your baby or not. It is at your 22 week scan that you get to make this decision, although some areas do not allow the sex of the baby to be revealed. Most hospitals will give you the choice of finding out if you want to though. I did with each of my children; I'm just too nosey to wait! If you would prefer the surprise then simply ask not to be told the sex, it's a personal preference so if you don't want to know beforehand tell them so, and you can find out on the day.

You may want to know to make sure you're on top of all the practicalities of the oncoming storm, such as what colour to paint the nursery and what colour pram to buy. Smaller decisions like the colour choice for clothes also plays a role as it is nice to have a little set of outfits at the ready for when baby makes an appearance, although it isn't vital. The range of neutral colours for all of these things is more than enough to put off making the decision if that is the only reason why you are doing so.

Getting Ready!

Given this trimester is the time when you will have the most energy, use it wisely. Make plans, write lists, and get anything you want accomplished before baby arrives done in the second trimester. As the third trimester comes a-knocking you will find your energy levels waning again and you'll regret not using your time wisely when you had the energy to do so.

Of course, you may not get the opportunity to do everything you want, and it just might be that what you want to get done simply has to wait. We were moving house during our third pregnancy, and what with surveys and completion dates being dragged out, we didn't complete until I was 7 months pregnant.

The hubby was away with work for a couple of months which meant I, and my 2 little helpers, had to move house pretty much by ourselves. In the evenings after work we would pack up a box or two before I'd collapse on the couch, and at weekends we'd pack some more. I think I progressively packed everything over the space of 4 weeks, though we also had the last minute rush to get everything done as well. How I managed to be so organised yet leave so many things to the last minute is beyond me!

I left finding a company who could clean the house until the last minute, meaning they couldn't do the date I needed before handing the house over, meaning I had to spend the day before the exchange day on hands and knees. If you have any similar jobs that need doing then make sure you schedule them in early as you don't want to be doing strenuous exercise in the last few months of pregnancy – I felt like I was going to pass out from exhaustion after simply hoovering the living room!

Don't rely on people to offer their help either, be forward about asking for assistance. Pride shouldn't be a factor in these things. I waited and waited for family and extended family to offer help moving but in the end had to ask for it. Don't feel cheeky as people won't view a request for help as cheekiness, unless you do it always.

Did You Know?

The umbilical cord is your baby's lifeline and the link between you and her/him. Your blood circulates through the cord, carrying oxygen and food to baby and carrying waste away from baby.

☐

Oooh, Matron: A Bit of Hanky Panky

As your stomach gets bigger and bigger, you may find your libido increasing. Don't be alarmed, this is natural. Women have reported feeling sexier and hornier during pregnancy than at any other time in their lives. I'm not sure why, maybe it's because it's impossible for us to get pregnant…again.

Either way, enjoy your new-found lust for love, and get your partner to indulge in a bit of hanky panky. Now, while some men will jump at this chance for more of the good stuff, some men may cower, nervous about the possibility of hurting the baby in some way.

It's incredible to realise that men still believe that they may hit the baby's head if they have intercourse. Re-assure them, it's just not possible. Sure, if you have had a difficult pregnancy or have experienced bleeding or stomach cramps, you may be advised against engaging in sexual intercourse, but if you are having a healthy pregnancy then there is no need to shy away from engaging in something that you would both enjoy.

Choosing a Name

A good way to while away a few hours is to get out a baby name book. It will probably take a few tries to agree on a name as it's a big decision. Before you choose something too wacky just remember that your baby is going to have this name for the rest of his/her life. Be kind. I've heard some really strange names, and my sister hated growing up with her unusual name. It's different when we're adults as we seek out things that make us unique, but when we're young we just want to be one of the group and shy away from the things that make us stand out.

It may be a shame but a lot of teasing starts out with names. That shouldn't make you change your mind if you fall in love with a certain name, but it is something to bear in mind if you just fancy something strange. My sister now loves the unusualness of her name but for years wished she was called something less original. It didn't help that it was a name that was difficult to shorten, which is something else you should bear in mind.

When choosing a name think about how the name can be twisted around by snotty kids, think about how the name goes with the surname and what the likely nickname will be as most kids do shorten names down.

Names that are popular at the moment seem to be harking back to an earlier age. Names that our grandparents had are now back in fashion, with William, Thomas, Alfie and Harry being popular amongst the boys and Lilly, Olivia, Emily and Jessica popular amongst girls.

TOP 5 BOY'S NAMES 2012
1. HARRY
2. JACK
3. CHARLIE
4. OLIVER
5. ALFIE

TOP 5 GIRL'S NAMES 2012

☐   AMELIA

☐   OLIVIA

☐   EMILY

☐   JESSICA

☐   SOPHIE

Get ready for lots of friendly arguments about names. The chances of agreeing on a name with your partner first time round is almost impossible. We all have favourite names, or names that we definitely do not want our children having. Choices are also limited by close relationships with other families. You may love a name but won't choose it for your child as your best friend or close relative has a child with the name. You may also love a name but have it vetoed by your partner as it was a name of an ex or they simply don't like it.

Some people choose their name almost immediately. Others wait until the baby is born, and others still find it really difficult to decide on the name and wait until registration day before finally agreeing on it. There is no right way or wrong way to choose your baby's name. If you agree on a name before the baby is born then so be it. Just be prepared to have a sudden change of heart as it is true what they say; once you meet your baby you may find that they do not suit their chosen name. That may sound foolish but you will know what I mean once you meet your little bundle of joy.

With our first child we batted names back and forth for months before finally agreeing on Jack. We waited until Jack was born before finally agreeing that was it, though if we'd decided he hadn't suited the name I'm not sure what we would have done as we couldn't agree on anything else.

With the other two we just couldn't decide. All the names we liked were names of children of close friends and relatives. We finally settled on their names a couple of hours after they were born.

A close friend struggled with a name for her child for so long it wasn't until the day she had to go and get the baby registered so the birth certificate could be produced that her and her partner finally settled on something.

This may be a bit mean but I really get annoyed by people who start referring to their baby by name whilst he/she is still in the womb. They will sign cards with their baby's new name on, send out invitations with their baby's name on and broadcast it to whoever will listen. What happens if you decide to change your mind after the baby is born, or is it so engrained in the subconscious at that point that the mere suggestion that the name doesn't fit the face would be a massive insult?

If you're struggling to refer to your baby as anything other than 'it' whilst your baby is still in your womb then try something generic like 'bump' or give it a cute name like 'button' or 'bunny'. Okay, instead of cute read corny.

Whatever name you decide on, whether it is months in advance, on the day of the birth or the day before you have to register the birth make sure you like it as you'll be calling it out for years to come.

Summary

I've given you enough hints that if you want to get anything done during your pregnancy, then the second trimester is the time to do it. This includes the last time your partner can whisk you away on a romantic holiday without having to co-ordinate with a list of other people and worry endlessly about childcare.

In your second trimester you should therefore:

- ➤ Get yourself ready for motherhood
- ➤ Organise your space and mind
- ➤ Enjoy your last taste of freedom
- ➤ Choose a Name and Decorate the Nursery
- ➤ Decide whether you want to know the sex of your child
- ➤ Have lots of sex

5 THE THIRD TRIMESTER

This is it, the home stretch. You're almost there! At 28 weeks your baby is perfectly formed, and now just needs to grow a bit more.

So you thought you were tired in the first trimester did you? Ha! Prepare to be exhausted! Climbing a flight of stairs? You might want to sit down for 5 minutes afterward. Going shopping? Allow for double the time – you will need lots of sit down breaks. And that doesn't mean coffee stops as you are not supposed to drink more than 3-4 cups a day. We live in a townhouse and I swear by the time I was on the second step of the second flight of stairs, I was huffing and puffing. Okay, I can't profess to being the fittest person in the world, but wow it takes it out of you!

Another thing, say goodbye to your bottom half. Cutting your toenails becomes a full hour task, with huffs and puffs for each nail. And don't even attempt to paint them as that will wear you out. And as for waxing or shaving or whatever it is you do, you'll need to use touch to decide whether you're in need or not as you won't be seeing anything.

Bending down becomes a slow chore and getting up from a crouching position requires some form of support, be it a helping hand or a cupboard door. You will start to feel pathetic and useless, and if you're anything like me, annoyed at the limited number of things you can get done before you need to sit down. This feeling only gets worse if you have kids already, as they won't understand that things you used to be able to do are now much more difficult and time consuming.

The number of appointments you now have to attend becomes a lot more restrictive as well, particularly if you are trying to work up to your due date as much as you possibly can. Just remember that no matter what, your employer is legally obliged to allow you to attend the myriad of appointments you will find yourself being booked in for. And be prepared to have a lot of blood taken. I seemed to have blood taken at almost every other appointment, although I have yet to learn my blood type (pathetic I know!).

Along with the kicking you start to see the actual movement in your third trimester. I was sitting watching tv in my parent's house one evening when the baby started doing its usual somersaults. My dad must have glanced over at that point as he exclaimed "what the hell was that!?" Yes Dad, I'm about to give birth to an alien who is going to leap out of my belly at any point – I'm pregnant, what do you think it is!? I assume it's just because the movement was so pronounced but the man was shocked.

I'm not entirely sure whether it's because it was so recent or whether I just can't remember the sensation of the other two, but I am sure this baby is the biggest kicker going. It is constantly on the move, rolling and kicking and stretching. I've even recorded video of my stomach so I can remember how much it moved about.

There are quite a few symptoms that you need to look out for in your third trimester. You may get swelling in your ankles or fingers, and many women find they have to remove their rings once they get into the third trimester as their fingers swell up. If your ankles or feet are prone to swelling consult your doctor to check everything is okay, and make sure you put your feet up regularly. I shouldn't need to tell you that you shouldn't be doing anything too strenuous and lifting is out of the question.

Also, whilst the saying goes "you're eating for two", it isn't technically true. True, you need to consume more calories, but not another 2000! And this is not an excuse to pig out on junk food (yes I know, I'm a right one to talk, what with my earlier confession about the chocolate!). Eat healthily, make sure you increase your intake of water and fresh fruit and vegetables, and make sure you take iron in some way, be it through some tasty burgers or through pregnancy supplements.

A lot of women get anaemic in the third trimester, myself included, so your doctor may prescribe iron tablets in addition to any other supplements you may be taking. This should help with any excessive tiredness you have been experiencing, although don't expect to suddenly come alive!

Another tip is to do pelvic floor exercises. There's nothing to them, and they do help. Simply pull in your "wee" muscles. Practice on the toilet if you must: mid flow simply try to stop weeing. Those muscles that you feel, they are the ones you want to exercise. And you can do it at any time, without anyone knowing. Just hold them in for 10 seconds at a time as many times as you want. If you find your muscles aren't as tight as they used to be i.e. a tiny bit of wee escapes when you sneeze or laugh, then you really need to do these as this can get worse once the baby comes if they are tightened.

Third Trimester Symptoms

You will begin to feel more and more tired. Lethargy took over my body in the later stages of pregnancy, and simple things like walking a flight of stairs left me huffing and puffing for about 5 minutes afterwards!

You may find it hard to sleep in the last trimester, particularly when heartburn kicks in and you are getting up to pee every couple of hours. If you're wondering what other wonderful symptoms or complaints you may face at this point then read on.

Backache

As your pregnancy progresses it is likely that you will experience significant discomfit, particularly in your lower back area. The problem is that your ligaments become softer and stretch to prepare your body for labour, straining the joints of your lower back and pelvis in the process.

There are a few things you can do to minimise the pain, such as:
- ➢ Avoid lifting heavy objects
- ➢ Bend your knees and keep your back straight when bending to pick something up from the floor
- ➢ Wear flat shoes
- ➢ Don't stoop
- ➢ Try to remain balanced i.e. don't carry all your shopping in one hand and leave the other free
- ➢ Check your posture
- ➢ REST

The 5th one might be a bit hard to do if you have older children, particularly if they are still toddlers and constantly want picked up!
The best advice I can give regarding back ache is to get a firm mattress. If that's not possible then put a piece of hardboard under your mattress to make it firmer. I remember my mum doing this when me and my sisters were kids.

Incontinence
Another common complaint is incontinence, which can affect you during your pregnancy as well as when your baby is born. Coughing, sneezing or laughing can result in a small amount of urine escaping and is mostly due to your pelvic floor muscles relaxing. Find exercises to tighten your pelvic floor muscles in the First Trimester section of this book.
Only 10 months after the birth of my son can I now sneeze without having to cross my legs before I do so. I never had incontinence on a grand scale but sneezing always used to trigger a tiny escape of wee. Another problem I had was when I really needed to go, sometimes I could barely control myself and had to race to the toilet before I had a little leakage. The glamorous side of pregnancy this stuff is not!

Indigestion and heartburn
For me, this one was my least favourite part of pregnancy, Yes, I had more than my fair share of least favourite parts but this one drove me mad. During my entire 3rd trimester with all 3 of my kids I would lie down in bed and indigestion would set in within minutes. As with everything else it's all down to hormones and your growing uterus pressing onto your stomach.
Apparently eating smaller meals can help, as can avoiding foods which seem to cause the indigestion, but in my experience, no matter what I did I couldn't get rid of it until the baby had arrived. Literally, the night after the

birth I lay down and just let out a sigh of relief: as if by magic, whoosh, and indigestion was no more.

If you're a fan of milk then try drinking a glass before bed as this has been known to help, otherwise prop yourself up with pillows. I hate milk, and my neck would start hurting after 10 minutes if I had more than one pillow under my head, so I couldn't shift the darn thing.

You can take antacids but you must check with your midwife or doctor before doing so.

Leaky nipples

One of my all-time favourites for the pure embarrassment of it! It's perfectly normal in the later stages of pregnancy for your nipples to leak, it just means your body is getting ready for the imminent birth of your child but, walking around with wet patches where you don't really want to have wet patches is not fun. Invest in some sexy breast pads, which you can pick up in the supermarket or at your local chemist/drugstore. Some just slot into your nursing bra whilst others have an adhesive patch so you can affix them to your clothing or normal bras. By the way, when I say sexy I really mean anything but!

Sleep

As if we weren't punished enough, in the last stages of pregnancy when you know you're about to spend the next few months waking up at every unearthly hour known to man, you'll find that you just can't get comfortable. Even better, when you do finally fall asleep you'll be up a couple of hours later needing to pee because the baby is lying on your bladder. You may also find yourself having really vivid dreams. I had some weird ones, too weird to mention here, suffice to say my husband found them very amusing, although the ones about death were just no fun.

Stretch marks

I spent the whole of my first pregnancy worrying about stretch marks. I'd heard horror stories, and as a result, religiously applied stretch mark cream every single night, and sometimes in the mornings too. Actually it was quite a fantastic ritual as for the first (and only) time my husband (who wasn't yet my husband but instead my mere fiancé) rubbed the cream into me almost every night, and would then read a story to his baby.

Very cute, I hear you say, but don't be fooled, by the time I was pregnant with the second I think I might have got a handful of creamy belly rubs, and by number 3 I just did it myself in a more slapdash manner. The romance was dead, might have had something to do with the fact that we got married after baby number 1.

Anyway, I digress, stretch marks are those pretty pink or purple lines which show up on your abdomen and sometimes even on your breasts and thighs. If you don't know what they look like imagine when you first got your boobies, if they were a good healthy size then odds are your skin stretched, and you got some nice stretch marks to boot. Sometimes they go, sometimes they don't. You're either lucky or you're not but chances are that if you put on lots of weight during your pregnancy you will probably get a nice set of stretch marks. Apparently the creams don't help but if you want to try them do. I did, and I was lucky enough to not get stretch marks with any of mine. Result!

Swelling joints
Your body retains more water during pregnancy and as the day wears on, and particularly if it's been a hot one or you've been standing a lot, the water gathers in the joints in your lower extremities, resulting in swollen feet, ankles and even fingers.
I didn't really get the swelling problem, I don't think I ever stood for longer than an hour, and that would have been throughout the whole day, okay maybe an hour and a half. My fingers did swell though, not noticeably but just enough so I couldn't wear my rings, which went down well with the hubby.
The answer to this problem is one of my favourites – rest. Try to rest with your feet up for at least an hour, do your foot exercises and don't stand for too long.
Another part of your body which can experience swelling is your veins, and the phrase for this is varicose veins. It's usually the veins in the legs that are affected but the veins in your vagina can also be affected. It's nothing to worry about and they should go soon after birth. To combat varicose veins don't stand for too long, exercise regularly as this will boost your circulation, don't sit with your legs crossed and try to maintain a healthy weight. If you are worried try sleeping with your legs higher than your body and make sure you do your foot exercises.

Other potentially more serious problems
Along with these common complaints and symptoms, there are some more serious problems which I'm just going to mention briefly. If you have any concerns about any of the problems I am about to mention then you should book in to see your doctor who can discuss your individual case.

High blood pressure and pre-eclampsia
Pre-eclampsia usually happens in the second half of pregnancy or immediately after birth and is thought to be due to a problem with the placenta and is linked to high blood pressure, fluid retention and protein in

urine. Your blood pressure and urine will be checked at every single antenatal check as high blood pressure and protein in your urine can be the first signs of pre-eclampsia. If left untreated pre-eclampsia can be life-threatening, this is why it is important to go for regular checks. Things to look out for are blurred vision, vomiting, pain below your ribs, severe headaches and sudden swelling of the hands or feet.

I always used to wonder why my blood pressure was taken at each and every check-up and I guess now I know why.

Placenta praevia

Placenta praevia is the medical name for a low lying placenta; when the placenta is near to or covering the cervix. The position of your placenta is checked at your 2nd ultrasound scan and if it is low you will be offered a 3rd scan when you are about 32 weeks pregnant. Usually the placenta corrects itself but if not you will be asked to go into hospital near your due date so you can be monitored as there is a higher chance of heavy bleeding, and you may also be offered a caesarean.

I had this with my 3rd child and didn't really understand it at all at first; they were so casual about it that I thought a 3rd scan was the new norm. It wasn't until I heard a hint of relief in the ultrasound technician's voice that I wondered whether they had been worried. All was good though and baby was born without any real problems.

Severe itching

This can be a sign of a condition called obstetric cholestasis which is a potentially dangerous liver disorder. The main symptom is severe itching in the second half of pregnancy. Don't be fooled by the simple sounding itching as this is an extremely serious condition and can lead to stillbirth or premature birth for baby and maternal haemorrhaging for mum. If your hands and feet become severely itchy or your skin starts to take on a yellow hue contact your doctor straightaway.

Bleeding

Bleeding during the early stages of pregnancy is very common, but what about the other 2 trimesters? Well, bleeding can happen after sex at any point of your pregnancy or it can happen as a result of a vaginal infection.

If you find blood near the end of your pregnancy then it will more than likely be the show, which is a mixture of blood and mucus which will tell you that your body is getting ready for labour. By now you should know what to do if you are worried (doctor).

Deep vein thrombosis

This serious condition can happen when a clot develops, usually in your legs, and becomes potentially life-threatening if it moves up to your lungs. The risks of developing this condition increase if you tend to sit still for long periods of time so make sure you regularly get up and walk about. If you are travelling on a long haul flight when pregnant then you should take precautions. Possibly invest in some flight socks and try to get up and have a walk up and down the aisles every hour or so.

And you will be pleased to know that that is the extent of the scary stuff I will be covering. Hopefully you experience none of the conditions mentioned above, and if you do I hope that it all turned out okay in the end and mum and baby were both healthy and happy.

TOP 5 ANNOYING PREGNANCY SYMPTOMS
- ➤ SICKNESS
- ➤ PILES
- ➤ STRETCH MARKS
- ➤ HEARTBURN
- ➤ TIREDNESS

The hospital bag

You should think about getting your hospital bag ready once you get to week 34 as you don't want to go into labour and then have to pack your bag.

Essentials for the bag are:
- ➤ A change of clothes for you to go home in
- ➤ Some comfortable clothes to wear during labour
- ➤ 2 outfits for baby: I would recommend a couple of vest tops and 2 sleepsuits.
- ➤ A handful of size 1 nappies
- ➤ Cotton wool balls
- ➤ Your wash bag as you will want to shower and freshen up after labour. Try to use sensitive creams and shower gels as you do not want anything that is overpowering or too scented.
- ➤ Underwear, either old ones or the throwaway maternity briefs
- ➤ Maternity towels
- ➤ Maternity bras and breast pads
- ➤ A towel, preferably a darker one as you will be bleeding
- ➤ You may want to take in pyjamas
- ➤ Some snack food for your birth partner and maybe even for you
- ➤ A TENS machine if you have hired/bought one
- ➤ A magazine or easy-to-read book
- ➤ Make sure you have the phone numbers of everyone you want to contact after the birth, as you may forget them on the day

As your pregnancy gets close to the end you will be more than ready for the baby to come. I think any woman you ask who is coming up to the 40 week milestone, or indeed has passed it, will say they just want their baby out now. With my third pregnancy, I was absolutely sick of heartburn, feeling uncomfortable, and being unable to do normal everyday activities without feeling exhausted.

Stocking Up

When you get home you will want to have the minimum amount to do that you possibly can. You will not want to be going out shopping. You will not want to be cooking big extravagant meals. You will not want to be socialising too much. What you will want to be doing is sleeping and cuddling your new bundle of deliciousness. Everything else just seems to fade into the background.

I read in countless books that I should cook up a storm before my due date and freeze down as much as I possibly could. As practical as this sounds, I'm not really a cook, and the idea of cooking enough of anything to freeze down fills me with horror. I've never frozen anything I've cooked. The reason for that is twofold: firstly, I never seem to make enough to freeze down, and even if I do make enough the hubby seems to see excess food and feel it his duty to eat just enough that it seems pointless to freeze the rest. Secondly, and I know this is rubbish, but I just don't fancy frozen down food. The hassle of taking it out and defrosting it, and what if it hasn't fully defrosted and how long can I keep it for and how do I reheat it? All these questions and no answers, so instead for the first few weeks we almost lived on takeaways and easy to make meals that John could buy in the local Tesco express and that took literally zero preparation time.

If you do like cooking then I would definitely advise you to pre-make as much as you can as you really do just feel drained. If you don't cook, or don't cook well, then just make sure you have lots of easy things in to make. Staples like pasta, couscous, rice can be bought way in advance as can the everyday things we need like toilet rolls, disinfectants and toiletries.

Your partner will have to get used to the idea of having to do the everyday shop for a little while. It won't kill them, and while you recover indoors and get used to your new role they can feel extremely useful by helping out in this way. If you are a single parent then ask a friend, family member or close neighbour to help you out for the first couple of weeks.

If you are lucky you may feel up to going out after a few days, particularly if the shops are within walking distance, but I would advise that you work on the premise that you won't want to go anywhere or do anything for a little while. Start with that and you'll surprise yourself when you start going stir crazy being cooped up indoors and have to escape.

One thing you will have to think about on your big shop before the due date is all the new stuff you will need to have in. Things like nappies, baby clothes, and cotton wool. Also remember for yourself you will need to have a wad of sanitary towels to hand as you will bleed quite heavily for a few days after labour. Think of it as your heaviest period ever and you should be fine. And make sure you buy the maternity pads, not the normal period stuff as the blood is significant in the first few days.

New parents are met with a mountain of choices when they first attempt the baby shop. What nappies should I buy? Do I need wipes? What am I missing? You need to have a clear idea in your head about how you want the first few weeks to go to enable you to do a proper shop.

Do you want to use disposable nappies or would you prefer to use eco-friendly nappies? Do you plan on breastfeeding or do you want to bottle feed straightaway? What toiletries do you need to buy for your baby?

To make it a tiny bit easier, I'd say forget baby toiletries for now as babies don't need anything in the way of toiletries. Water is all you need to clean them in their first few weeks. Even when they are older you shouldn't use too much product, keep it simple and as natural as possible.

Nappies you will need. And lots of them! Whilst I don't want to go into the trials and tribulations of early parenthood – we'll save that one for another day – I do want to touch on the first few things you will need to consider, and although you may think so little of it now, your brand choice on nappies will come to be your all-encompassing dilemma at least once in the first 12 months of parenthood.

Everyone does it. They decide on a brand, then hear from a friend about another brand that's far better than the one they're using, so they swap. Sometimes the change works and sometimes it doesn't. I religiously stuck to Pampers and Huggies with my firstborn. I tried to deviate from the path with my second son and mixed it up with some supermarket-brand nappies (read diapers if you are reading this over the pond). I also tried some nappies from a chemist. The supermarket-brand nappies brought Joe out in a nasty rash, literally within 24 hours of using the nappies his skin was raw and blotchy. I never used them again. The chemist bought nappies just couldn't hold up to the amount of night-time peeing activity they were seeing.

It wasn't until my 3rd child that I decided to give a different supermarket brand a try. This time it worked, and I use the same brand on my 2nd son, who had such a bad reaction to the other supermarket brand the first time round.

The reason why I'm telling this fascinatingly dull story is to show that brand allegiance isn't always a good, and isn't always a bad thing either. If you try a brand and are happy with it then stick with it. If you want to try a different brand then just buy a small pack of nappies as they may not suit. And just because a particular brand works fantastically for one family, it doesn't mean it's going to work the same way for yours.

A lot of the decision making about the brand choice is taken by the price, which can differ drastically between the leading name brands and the basic range at your local supermarkets. Try a few of the lower value brands as they will often work just as well as the leading brands.

It should go without saying but the same philosophy applies to wipes. Don't buy the most expensive ones unless you really like them, and don't be put off by the cheaper ones as they do still work. I tend to go for the fragrance-free ones which seem as natural as possible.

I have to confess to loving baby wipes. Who knew how many different things they could be used for? I use them to wipe clean my coffee table on a daily basis, clean the kids' faces after they've eaten, wipe down table surfaces after play and have even been known to use one to clean school shoes when in a hurry. I honestly can't imagine a time when I will stop buying them. It won't be for the next 8 years at any rate. And like nappies you can always find some on offer.

Whilst I love baby wipes, I don't use them on newborns, and you will be advised not to as well by your midwife. If you think about the stuff baby wipes are effective at removing, I've been known to get pen marks and wine stains out using baby wipes, then you'll guess that they can't be the best thing for baby's skin, as new as it is. For the first few weeks at least you should try and use water and cotton wool balls. I admit it's a lot more time-consuming and messy than just grabbing the pack of wipes but for the sake of a couple of extra minutes who cares!? Your baby's skin will thank you.

The Build Up

In the back of mind I really wanted a home birth for my third pregnancy. I think there's something romantic and wonderful about being able to give birth at home, amongst your own personal space. But the practicalities of it for me far outweighed the romanticism of the venture. First, where would we put the paddling pool? Second, how would we get it blown up and ready in time and more importantly, how would we clean it up and get it back down again? What about the other 2 kids? How would that work? If the labour started at 4am in the morning could we honestly expect the grandparents to drive over, pick up the boys and take them back to their house?

The only thing I knew was that I didn't want them there when I was giving birth. Who needs the added stress of that? In no way do I get anyone saying they'd like their other children involved in the birth, and in no way would I have liked to be involved in the birth of any of my siblings. I don't need them harassing me, or watching on in horror as I scream blue merry murder.

As such, we prompted for a hospital birth. As we'd recently moved areas I didn't get time to scope out all the options, and never even had a hospital visit so I could be shown around the maternity suite. I would definitely recommend doing this as the visits are usually run by one of the midwives who will be able to show you what will happen, where you will go and how events will likely take place. You will also get to check out the rooms and facilities on offer, such as the birthing pools. Not something for you to worry about, but definitely one for the partner is the parking situation. Paying a visit to the hospital beforehand will alert you to any potential problems you may face on the day, i.e. will you have to drive through a busy town centre location or is there enough adequate parking and will you need lots of coinage to pay for parking?

Another nice thing about going on the hospital tour is that you will meet other expectant parents who will all usually be due around the same time as you, so may even start up some much needed friendships with other new mums. Even if you have a fantastic group of mates already, it is nice to be able to share things with people who are going through the exact same stages as you. My advice would be to remain open to the possibility of new friendships, what's the harm in befriending another pregnant woman, who couldn't benefit from a new friend or two?

Of course, what I advise and I what I actually do are two different things altogether. Through 3 pregnancies, across 3 different hospitals, and we didn't attend one maternity ward open event. The first time wasn't our fault. We had the tour booked in, but baby came 5 ½ weeks early so we were actually there when our tour group was going round.

Whether you choose to spend your labour in a hospital, midwife-led centre or at home it is completely up to you. The best thing you can do is to write all your wants and wishes down in your birth plan.

Did You Know?

Inside your uterus, your baby is floating in a bag of fluid called the amniotic sac. Before or during labour the sac, or 'membranes', break and the fluid drains out. This is what we know as your 'waters breaking'.

What is a birth plan and when should I write one?

A birth plan is a record of what you would like to happen during your labour, such as do you want pain relief medication early on? Do you want to have a water birth? Do you want an epidural? Your birth plan should reflect what you want your labour to look like, taking into account any existing medical history. For example, you may want a home birth but if you have a pre-existing medical condition then a home birth would be ruled out and you would usually be required to attend hospital for your birth.

You should discuss your birth plan with your midwife and talk through options to make sure that your request is, firstly, medically safe and secondly is viable. Your birth plan might be extremely similar to your friend's or it may be completely different as each plan should be tailored to the individual.

Keep a copy of your birth plan and take it with you when you go in to give birth. The midwives will discuss your plan and try as much as they can to stick to it. However, don't be surprised if things don't go exactly as you've written. Birth plans are a good starting point but labours never go smoothly and the chances of you having to divert from your original plans are strong. This is why you should consider things like whether you want pain medication or whether you want to try to have a natural birth.

There is absolutely nothing wrong with getting so far into your labour and deciding you want to go off script. Maybe you wanted to go all natural but once the pain starts you may decide it is time for drugs of some sort, be that gas and air or an epidural. You may be in labour for so long the midwives may advise that you have a caesarean, and undoubtedly that would not have been in an all-natural birth plan, but circumstances change and you have to do what's best for baby and you.

Take the advice of the midwives if you feel comfortable with it as they certainly know what they are talking about, and will have been through similar situations a lot more times than you or I. Try not to get too stressed if things don't go according to plan and just think about what you will have when it's all over.

My labour stories
I really wanted to have a water birth, and by the third pregnancy thought it's now or never as I had missed the opportunity at both of my other births. The first one had been too early, and I had been hooked up to monitors, checking the baby's health and making sure nothing untoward was happening.

That labour took 9 hours once the contractions really kicked in, and there must have been about 6 people in the room when I finally gave birth. It was a teaching hospital so I had a bunch of students checking out what was going on. Now you may think, I would never allow that, and I would have been right there with you. However, once you're in that much pain you really just don't care who sees what, you just want it over with.

I had an episiotomy that time round, which is a tiny cut they make if the baby needs more room to get out. If you have a choice between getting an episiotomy or waiting to see if you tear then I would say go for the episiotomy. Of course it's personal preference, and your midwife would probably disagree with me strongly!

My second time round I tore in the exact same spot (apparently) and the natural tear hurt a heck of a lot more, and took longer to heal. To say I could actually feel the tear happening is no lie.

I was so very very happy when I came through my third labour with no tear at all, and boy did I notice the difference in the aftermath. It took only a few days to be able to walk around okay whereas the second time round it stung for 2 weeks.

They don't tell you about the stinging sensation afterward, and the uncomfortable sitting and standing you have to endure. But if you think that's bad then consider the after effects of a caesarean, where you are advised not to drive or lift anything heavy for at least 6 weeks, and you have an itchy stomach for months afterwards.

Saying that, I was talking with a friend about her labour as she had had a second caesarean and she admitted that the second time around she felt almost back to normal after only 2 weeks. Obviously that isn't going to happen with everyone, but it just shows that everybody is different and our bodies work in wondrous ways.

When I was first pregnant I created a template for my birthing plan. You may guess that my job at the time was creating documents and managing spread sheets. It may have seeped into my personal life, or I may have had a spare hour twiddling my thumbs at my desk.

My original birth plan stated that I wanted a water birth. I've always fancied the idea of giving birth in the water. I don't know why, I can't even swim! I remember reading somewhere that it was less stressful for the baby as they go from the amniotic fluid-filled sac inside your womb to the fluid-like water of the birthing pool rather than a brightly-lit sterile hospital room.

Suffice to say that I didn't get my water birth first time round. Second time round I was adamant I wanted that water birth. However, I turned up at the hospital in labour already. My contractions had been hardly anything when I phoned the parents at 8:00am to come and collect my eldest before the husband drove me into hospital. I vividly remember the hubby asking if I wanted anything to eat – if you can face eating I would do so as you won't get anything once you're at the hospital and it could be hours before your next meal. I had a fried egg sandwich. It was delicious.

We got to the hospital a little after 09:30 and it took us about 20 minutes to park up and walk over to the maternity unit. By this point (the walk was about 10 minutes but felt like 40!) the contractions were coming in stronger and stronger. We had to catch a lift up to the second floor and I remember a woman in the lift looking horrified as I stepped in, and exclaiming "I can't be in a lift with a pregnant woman". I felt like shouting "then get the hell out!" but a contraction kicked in as I opened my mouth. Would that be the first time my baby would stop me doing something stupid? No doubt it wouldn't be the last.

We made it to the maternity unit and I declared I was desperate for the toilet, which was conveniently located next to the front desk. The hubby stayed at the desk to complete the paperwork and hand over my folder. I had an overwhelming feeling of needing to poop but as I sat down I realised it was a little more than that, I wanted to push.

I screamed out to the hubby "I'm pushing!" and next thing the door swung open and a midwife had a wheelchair in there. I half-sat in the chair and was whisked through to a delivery suite and a mere 25 minutes later my second son was born.

No water birth. No time to discuss anything about a birth plan. The midwives were happy because it was nice and easy. I was not. As I was pushing I felt the tear burning through my skin. It was horrendous. I promised myself right then and there that I would never have another child. Ever.

We hadn't even agreed on a name and so, ever romantic, we discussed names as I was sewn up by a student midwife. A slow and painful experience in itself. We chose Samuel, and I was ecstatic at how small and immaculate and wonderful he was.

I was also a little gutted that I didn't get to experience the water birth. Moving on to pregnancy number 3... Yes I know I was adamant about the whole "never-having-another" thing but who doesn't say that mid-labour!?

Third time round and this was it. Water birth here I come. As soon as we got to the hospital I made it clear that I wanted a water birth and they were very nice about it as well.

We went in when the contractions were still quite gentle so I envisaged a cup of tea, maybe a snack, walk around and then go in to the birthing pool area. What happened went slightly against plan.

We arrived at the maternity ward only to be told I had probably come in too early and should go back home. This made me a little nervous given how fast Samuel had come, but I relented.

First though, they offered to show us the midwife-led unit, which was much nicer and used by low risk women. It was definitely much nicer, the rooms were newly painted, as opposed to the ones in the maternity ward, which were chipped and cracked and multi-coloured.

You got your own private room for the duration of your stay, with en-suite. It felt almost private it was that nice. At this point, I want to say one thing: we may moan about it a lot, but the NHS is an amazing thing. Both Americans and Australians have to actually pay for the privilege of giving birth and here we are getting it for free, and getting very comfortable doing so. I love the NHS, it is an amazing thing that we take for granted far too often.

Anyway, back to it: the unit was lovely. The midwife said I could go home she just wanted to check with the midwife in charge that I was okay to come back to the unit once I came in for real. Thankfully the midwife in charge, on hearing about my second labour, suggested I hang around and go for a walk around the hospital.

It took 15 minutes of walking. I left the unit quite bubbly and personable. 15 minutes later I staggered back in, fully supported by the hubby at this point, panting and moaning.

"You look a bit different to when you left" the midwife smiled. She promised she'd be with us in 30 minutes and sent us to our room.

Whilst roaming the hospital corridors, as the contractions started getting more severe, I stopped about 4 times, clinging onto the railings and gritting my teeth against the pain. Each time I did this I noticed the hubby cringing with embarrassment, and at one point even trying to move me along. Every part of my being wanted to swop bodies with him just for 5 minutes so he could experience what I was experiencing, then he wouldn't have given 2 hoots about what anyone was thinking. We were in a hospital after all; if you're going to be walking past people in pain you can't really complain about it can you!

Getting back to my room I tried to get comfortable on the bed but couldn't. How can you get comfortable when your whole body is getting ready to push a person out of you!? 10 minutes passed, maybe it was 20 I have no idea but I know it felt much longer. The midwife popped her head through the door, "just checking you're okay, and I'll be with you shortly" she said before turning to leave.

I shouted out, "No, you can't go" before breaking into another contraction. After explaining that I really wanted to push she checked "down there" and confirmed that I was much further along than she thought I would be.

I demanded gas and air and was close to tears when I realised 5 minutes after getting it that the thing was broken. That I gave labour with no pain relief at all was a travesty as far as I was, and still am, concerned. Gas and air got me through 2 labours and now all I had was the hubby rubbing my back and stroking my hair. Rubbish!

When I realised 4 people were surrounding my lower body area and talking with concerned looks on their faces I started getting nervous.

When the main midwife told me to push and keep pushing until I couldn't push anymore I didn't know whether to push or cry. When I told her I couldn't do it anymore and needed a break and she told me I didn't have any other option but to push I just didn't know how I was going to muster up enough energy to keep going.

No-one tells you how exhausting it is pushing out a baby. It winds you. It tires you. It hurts like hell; I'm not going to lie. I tried a scream when I next pushed and was shouted at for wasting energy on screaming. "Just push, concentrate everything you have on pushing". And so I pushed. And pushed again. And pushed again, until I felt something come out and everyone jump into action before a collective sigh echoed around the room. Little had I known but my baby had the cord wrapped around his neck and had been struggling to breathe. He was fine though, better than fine, he was gorgeous. And he was the only one who went straight for the nipple and had his first proper suck no more than 5 minutes after coming out. The hungry Horace!

Scary things happen in labour, but what I learnt from my scary experience is to trust the experience in the room. If your midwife says you must do something I'd do what she says. Sometimes they can be a bit harsh but I guess at times they need to be. The only thing that mattered to me was that my baby was okay, and for that I have the midwives to thank. I hate to think what could have happened if I had gone home.

Why do you think women like to tell their labour story to others? Because it's so personal! No two stories will ever be the same. Your story belongs to you and no-one else would be able to replicate. Heck even you probably wouldn't replicate it as next time round your labour will probably be different in some way to the first time.

If you are lucky enough you may get to go home on the same day, although you may have to stay if you give birth later on in the day as hospitals must keep you in for 5 hours from birth as procedure. If you do have to stay over and it is in a nice ward then just lie back and enjoy the extra help for the night. The midwives will be able to give you advice on latching on and getting started with breastfeeding, they can also show you how best to bathe your baby and discuss any other concerns you may have. If you have had an extremely long and hard labour they may even offer to watch your baby for a couple of hours while you get some sleep, but of course that is dependent upon staffing levels and how busy the ward is. At the very least you will get dinner, lunch and/or breakfast and will be able to settle back in bed and not start worrying about too much too soon.

If you've already got children at home you may want to just get home to be with your family, then again you may welcome the chance for one-on-one time with your new-born before you enter the chaos of home.

With my eldest I ended up staying in hospital for 10 days. It was horrific. We were both fine but as Jack had been born so early he was tiny – 5lb 10oz. We wouldn't be allowed home until he could put weight on over 2 consecutive days.

The second day I felt fine and wondered why some of the mums were weepy. One of the midwives explained that by day 5 the mums got all emotional and fed up with being cooped up in the hospital. I felt sorry for them and thought it was such a shame that they felt sad, but knew I wouldn't feel that way – I was made of tougher stuff.

So you know what happened next right? Yep, day 5 I was a mess. The hubby's parents came in to see Jack and hubby stepped out of the ward to take a call. John's mum asked some mundane question, I don't even remember what it was, and I suddenly found myself sobbing. John's Dad quickly made his excuses and escaped to hunt down John. I didn't really have any reason for feeling upset, it just suddenly started and then I couldn't stop it. Maybe it was being cooped up for so long, maybe it was hormones, I have no idea.

Whatever it was it must have had some impact on the in-laws as 2 days later they came in and sat with Jack while John took me to the hotel next door to have a tasty meal. I only had tomato soup but I remember it being the best food I'd tasted in ages. After hospital food for 5 days I'm not surprised!

It didn't sink in until I had my second son but the hospital setting can be so important. With my first child I gave birth in a hospital that was pretty dilapidated. Most of the hospital had been shut and there was only a few departments left, maternity being one of them. They were in the process of building a new hospital but that wouldn't be finished for another 2 years.

It was depressing with long empty corridors and an overwhelming sense of being somewhere lost in time. One good thing about the hospital was that they had a special transition ward for women and babies in a similar situation to my own. Without that ward Jack would have been taken to a special baby unit so I am definitely thankful for that. What I am not thankful for was the size of the ward – there were 16 beds in the 1 ward, all occupied with women and their babies.

Some of the women would be there for just a day or two, others like me were there for a week or more. Some of the babies were of a similar size to Jack and some were almost twice the size.

There was a kitchen a short way down the corridor where we could help ourselves to tea and toast and baby milk. I had a horrible time those first couple of weeks, trying to breastfeed. Jack was too weak to latch on properly so they encouraged me to express with an electric double pump. It took me about 30 minutes to express 2 ounces, it was pathetic. What was even more disheartening was that some women could express a full 9 ounces in a matter of minutes.

I felt like I went from expressing to trying to feed back to expressing. As there were only two electric expressers on the ward you had to wait your turn to use them, and would always have someone waiting behind you, just to add another level of pressure. I hated it and almost gave up with the whole breastfeeding thing.

Jack was given my milk – he had to be fitted with a tube as he was so weak - but had to be topped up with formula milk as I couldn't produce enough. It was soul-destroying, especially as I had wanted to breastfeed so much. If it wasn't for an older midwife who did the night shift and who encouraged me to keep trying I would have moved Jack exclusively onto formula. As it was she showed me some techniques I could use and convinced me to persevere.

Whilst there were some amazing midwives, don't think that every single one is like that. I encountered a couple of right snooty cows. There was one woman who practically screamed at a new mum who had gone through a similar experience to my own and moved her baby onto formula milk, and there was a young mum who was constantly berated for feeding her baby formula food. I think we all know how amazingly beneficial breast milk is, but if a mum is that much against breastfeeding I don't think she should be made to feel like a villain because of her choices.

When you're thinking about your birth plan think seriously about where you want to have your baby, and visit more than one place. Not that it would have mattered due to giving birth prematurely, but if I'd have gone to the hospital beforehand I wouldn't have wanted to make that my first choice.

The hubby had to complain to staff after day 5 of being in the hospital when I was still sitting on the same blood-soaked pad as they had given me on day 2. He also had to ask them to change the sheets – again blood-stained.

One time he draped his coat on the bottom of my bed. It fell off onto the floor and when he picked it up it was covered in dust. It may come as no surprise then that the young mum next to me contracted MRSA, as did her baby, and both had to be moved to a private room for the remainder of their stay.

Do you think the staff then disinfected the ward to ensure no further risk? No. They cleaned the tiny little cubicle space. They didn't even come near me and for the life of me I can't remember ever seeing my area cleaned, disinfected or even wiped. Hospital standards certainly aren't what they used to be.

Saying that, the second and third hospitals were both immaculate compared to that first one. And yes, I had my babies in a different hospital each time as we moved around between each birth.

One thing I recommend if you also find yourself stuck in the hospital for a few days is to get your partner to kit you out with comfy pjs, bring in loads of mindless magazines for you to leaf through and lots of snacks and goodies. You will be tireder than you've ever felt before, or at least I was, and couldn't have read anything heavier than a gossipy magazine.

John used to come in every afternoon laden with crusty bread, a variety of cheeses, grapes, apples, chocolate milkshake and chocolate biscuits. The midwives told me that the best way to bring in my milk was to pig out on lots of dairy, and I wasn't about to complain! As well as eating more dairy than I have in a long time I also got through a massive amount of hot chocolate. I stopped short of adding whipped cream each time, but I did indulge sometimes. And whenever I'd had one of these naughty suppers I'd have a go at expressing more milk, and it usually worked a lot better than when I'd express after the boring hospital food. Not sure whether that was more mind control rather than me eating the "right" stuff but it worked for me.

John also smuggled in MacDonald's and takeaway Chinese to rescue me from the horrors of the hospital food. Rescuing me from the horrors of sharing a room with 30 other people was a little harder. If it wasn't your own child crying then invariably someone else's child would keep you up while they screamed for whatever it was they needed. Add to that the helpful midwives who would wake you religiously for the nappy change or feed time. Often I'd just get to sleep when I'd be woken up to prepare for the next feed. I couldn't wait to get home.

Every day I'd dread and look forward to the weigh in with equal measure. Whilst Jack would put a tiny bit of weight on one day he would always lose it the next. By the 10th day I had my fingers and toes crossed that he would put a bit more weight on, and he finally did. The midwife agreed to speak to the doctor and assured us that we would finally be able to go home. I've never been so happy.

John on the other hand was frantic. Whilst I had been laid up in a hospital bed going stir crazy for the last 10 days he had been trying to get the house ready for us coming home. He had done all the Christmas shopping – Jack arrived on 12th December – and had even found time to put up a Christmas tree and decorate our living room. A less glamorous task was cleaning our mattress.

When I was 6 months pregnant we had bought a new bed as I had started getting really bad backache and was advised that a firmer mattress would do the trick. It did help massively, but our lovely new bed was ruined on the night I went into labour, when my waters broke all over the bed.

I woke up feeling wet and sticky with a horrible stench pervading my nostrils – no-one tells you that your waters have a distinctively masculine smell, if you catch my drift. Yep, I swear it smells of sperm. Or is that just me? Anyway, I waddled across the hallway to the bathroom, leaving John in bed whilst I worried about whether I'd wet myself or not.

Whilst I was in the bathroom cleaning myself up, John had woken to find himself in bed alone, also wet. He confessed that the first thought that had gone through his head was that he had wet the bed and I, disgusted, had gone into the other room. When I waddled back in and told him I think my waters had broken he thought I had gone mad.

We called the hospital delivery suite and they advised that we come straight in due to the fact that it was over a month earlier than it should have been. John, being the kind and considerate man that I knew him to be, decided he needed some food first and made some fried egg sandwiches before putting on the tv to watch the boxing match. Charming! I got dressed and we finally set off for the hospital – once the boxing match had finished of course! Thankfully it was a pretty short one or I would have been furious.

I didn't really have any stomach contractions at first with my first labour. It was more like intense back spasms. We got to the hospital and they checked me over, and advised me to stay the night just to be sure everything was okay. They were going to give me something to try and delay labour.

John went home to get some sleep and I promised to call if anything further happened. At this point it was about 7am in the morning and all I wanted to do was sleep. The breaking waters had happened at 2am and we'd only got to bed at 12:30 so I was shattered.

I tried to go to sleep but I kept having intermittent pains in my back, and when the midwife came over to check on me she felt my stomach and confirmed that I was indeed in labour. All I could think about was the fact that I still hadn't had any sleep and I really wanted to get some before I had to deal with labour and a baby.

No such luck. John was called back and we were moved downstairs into one of the delivery suites. Across the hallway I could hear someone in the throes of labour, screaming shrilly. It sounded horrendous. I just wanted to go back upstairs to bed.

Once labour started in full, about 2 hours later, one of the midwives came in to announce my mum and dad had arrived to visit. They'd known we'd come into the hospital, and that I had been advised to stay overnight, but not that it had progressed quickly and we had gone into labour. Rather than send them away without even a hello I told the nurse to let my mum in to say hello. She ended up staying for the duration and after me and the hubby, was the next person to see our new arrival (apart from the doctors and nurses of courses).

Having my mum there allowed the hubby to step out and have a break every so often. I didn't learn until later that when he was stepping outside to take a break he was secretly being fed hot, buttery toast and tea by the midwives.

Labour

They say you will know when you go into labour, but in my experience it isn't that simple. No-one knows what labour feels like until they've experienced it, though the 2nd and 3rd time round I knew straightaway. First time round though you may wonder how you will know you are going into labour, I certainly did.

You may have a couple of false alarms as you work up to the day, and some women suffer from something called Braxton Hicks contractions, which can be described as practice contractions, as your body gets ready for its biggest challenge to date. When your contractions do start in earnest you should know, the big clue will be the massive pains you will experience, though if you read my first labour experience you'll know it isn't always that clear cut.

If you find yourself standing in a big, or little, puddle of water though, you can be pretty sure your waters have broken, unless you knowingly peed yourself. Once your waters break it's only a matter of time before labour starts.

Another good indication of the impending pain is what they call the "show", which is a ball of blood and goopy stuff that will likely come out a few days before labour starts. The "show" is the plug of mucus in the cervix, which comes away as your body starts to ready itself for labour. The mucus plug helped to seal the uterus during pregnancy and while it contains a bit of blood, if you are worried about the amount of blood that you see then call your midwife or the hospital straightaway as there should not be too much to overly concern you.

Another symptom of labour is backache – my one overriding symptom during my first labour. It may feel like a dull ache or a heavy feeling, and can feel akin to the backache you may experience during your monthly period.

The other symptom that I experienced first throughout each labour was my waters breaking. Your "waters" is actually a bag of water surrounding your baby which breaks just before labour is due to start. Waters breaking can either mean a slow and uncontrollable trickle or a sudden gush of water. Both are uncontrollable and both can happen at any time so don't be embarrassed when it does.

When your waters break take it as your cue to phone your midwife. If you have had a normal pregnancy and everything is on schedule your midwife may suggest you stay at home before the contractions really kick in, but if you have had other symptoms, your waters break early or you have had any complications then you may be advised to go straight to the delivery suite for assessment.

If you're wondering what a contraction is it is the uterus tightening up and then relaxing. At first the contractions will be short and will be spaced out 10 minutes or more, but as your labour proceeds the contractions will get stronger, last longer and come more quickly.

As part of your birth plan you will, or should, have discussed pain relief with your midwife and your birthing partner. Don't worry if you suddenly decide you want to deviate from your chosen path. If you want gas and air, then simply ask. Don't feel like you have to do it all completely naturally if you are feeling the pain. The drugs are there to help so don't be afraid to ask.

So what kind of pain relief will be on offer? You've got a few choices. The first one is termed self-help and involves techniques that you can use to help you cope with the pain. You may use deep breathing techniques, such as the breathing exercises you use in yoga, to relax and calm yourself. Deep breathing techniques can also help to focus your mind and may even help you to control the pain, or work through the contractions.

Moving around can also help with the pain. Try bouncing on one of the big birthing balls, or rocking back and forth. Walk around the room or if you are bed bound try changing positions, and kneeling against the pillows or lying on your side for a little while.

I made my husband rub my back for hours during my first labour. It helps! He complained of tired wrists for days afterwards but it does relieve some of the tension that builds up around your pelvis.

Try setting up a playlist for your labour. You may want to choose songs that relax you and make you smile or you may want to choose upbeat songs that will give you more energy and provide some much-needed motivation. Remember that music is one of the most powerful mediums available to us, and if you don't believe me try watching one of your favourite film clips without the soundtrack and see whether you get the same emotional reaction.

Having a bath can help relax you, and make the contractions seem less painful, but don't use bubble bath or other perfume-related goodies. If you want to use essential oils ask a qualified holistic therapist which ones are suitable as some are not recommended during pregnancy and will be a definite no-no during labour.

If you do find yourself relaxing to the smell of lavender then try a candle or an oil burner in your room, though you'll want to keep them away from your immediate area in case you knock them over.

Definitely my favourite pain relief choice is the gas and air, professionally known as Entonox. I used this during all 3 of my deliveries, though it ran out pretty soon into my 3rd labour, which caused me no end of anguish! This option doesn't get rid of the pain, but it does make it easier to bear and it's easy to use. You can use as little or as much as you want, just keep it away from your birth partner, who will undoubtedly want to try some themselves. I don't know what it is about men and gas and air but I've not met one yet who hasn't given it a go whilst in the delivery room, or maybe I just know the wrong type of men!

If you do choose to use gas and air then you will be given a mouthpiece which you hold. As your contraction begins you will want to inhale the gas using the mouthpiece. The gas takes only seconds (about 20) to work and works best if inhaled slowly and deeply. Word of warning though, don't inhale too much as it can make you queasy and very nauseous. If at any time you decide you don't like it then you can simply stop using it and the effects will quickly wear off.

Another non-invasive pain relief method is the TENS machine. TENS stands for Transcutaneous Electrical Nerve Stimulation. During your antenatal classes you will usually be given the option to hire a TENS machine, although you can also buy them from most pharmacies if you would prefer that option.

The way it works if you want to hire one is that they work on your due date. They give you a machine for a 2 week period usually, that straddles either side of your due date. You can request to keep it for longer if you over run your due date but if you come early, like I did, then basically – TOUGH! I was gutted my first time round that I didn't get the TENS machine, and I think given that most of my contractions felt like they were happening in my back I would have found it really useful. However, I didn't even bother the 2nd and 3rd time round, pure laziness and nothing more.

The main benefit you will get from the TENS machine is during the early stages of labour when you are more likely to experience lower back pain, but as your labour progresses it will become less and less effective.

The TENS machine sends little pulses of current through your body, stimulating it to produce more endorphins, which are your body's natural painkillers. The machine does this through the electrodes that you tape onto your back. These electrodes are connected by wires to a small battery-powered stimulator known as an 'obstetric pulsar'. Using a TENS could also reduce the number of pain signals your brain is sent by your spinal cord. There are no known side effects so it is a very safe form of pain relief.

If you want anything stronger you will be looking at using intramuscular injections, such as pethidine or diamorphine. I never had injections so have no experience of them or their side effects, but many friends used them to relieve pain. They take about 20 minutes to work and can last for between 2 to 4 hours.

Your midwife will not administer this form of pain relief if you are close to delivering your baby as they can interfere with your baby's breathing and make it difficult to push when you need to. Pethidine or diamorphine can also make you feel sick and forgetful and can interfere with breastfeeding.

If you are experiencing a particularly painful labour or a very long labour you may be asked if you would like an epidural. An epidural is a special type of anaesthetic which can only be administered by an anaesthetist. It numbs the nerves that carry pain from the birth canal to your brain and can offer complete pain relief.

If you choose to have an epidural you will have a drip inserted into a vein in your arm, then you will be asked to lie on your side or sit in a curled up position while the anaesthetist numbs a small area of your back. A small tube will be inserted into your back near the nerves that carry the pain and the drugs are administered through this tube. It takes about 20 minutes to set up an epidural and a further 15 minutes for the effects to be felt. Once set up the epidural can be topped up by either the anaesthetist or midwife, or even by yourself in some cases. Your contractions will be continuously monitored if you choose this option and as such you will have to wear a belt around your abdomen and potentially your baby will have to have a clip attached to its head.

Depending on the type of epidural you have your legs may feel very heavy and the second stage of your labour can be prolonged. Your midwife will probably have to tell you when you need to push as you may lose some sensation, and instruments may be needed to help deliver your baby, such as forceps.

The side effects of having an epidural include difficulty passing water, developing a headache, getting pins and needles down your leg after baby is born or experiencing back pain for a couple of days after childbirth. All these side effects are temporary and should go after a day or two.

If you choose not to use conventional pain relief then you may choose to go down the holistic route. There are a few options open to you, including hypnosis, aromatherapy, massage and reflexology. If you do choose to use one of these options then make sure you discuss your choices with your midwife who will be able to advise you how best to incorporate your wishes into your birth plan.

If you just want to get it over and done with then the best advice I've been given is to simply walk around. It worked with both my younger boys, and I'm positive all that walking around the hospital corridors led to my quick deliveries. So the best tip I can give is: keep moving. This does not mean massive exercise routines, but gentle walks and using the birth balls to rock back and forth.

Now you're in labour, what exactly happens?
There are 3 stages to labour. First, you dilate. Second, you give birth. Third, you push out the placenta.

First stage of labour – dilation
This is when the cervix starts opening up, or dilating. Your cervix needs to open up to about 10cm for your baby to come out; this is what is termed "fully dilated". Your contractions are the movements that soften your cervix and open it up and this process can takes hours. When your cervix is open to 4cm you are termed as being in "established labour". At this stage you could be pushing for a good few hours before you reach this milestone.

If you are not in established labour you may be advised to go back home. Make sure you eat, drink and rest as you are going to need all the energy you can get. Labour is exhausting, and just when it's finished and you need to rest, you have a newborn baby who is going to need you more than anyone or anything else has ever needed you before.

Again, if you do nothing else before labour, REST!! Trust me; you'll even forget what the word means after the first few weeks of blissful sleeplessness.

Once you've rested up, and if you are getting restless, you can walk around and keep active to progress your labour. Moving around will help your cervix to dilate and help move the baby down into your pelvis.

Once you are in established labour you will be checked regularly. If you're unsure what that would feel like or unsure when you need to go back to the hospital, a good indicator is the length of your contractions, and time between contractions. If the time between your contractions come down to 5 minutes then you want to be scooting off to the delivery suite pretty darn fast.

TIP: Get your birthing partner to drive the route to the hospital a couple of times so they know exactly where they are going. Know where to park the car and have enough change in the car to see you through a few hours at the minimum. Know where the closest doors are, and where the delivery suite is in the hospital. We didn't do any of these things with our 2nd son and regretted it as soon as we pulled up to the hospital as we had no idea where we were going. We had to ask about 3 different people before we finally found the delivery suite, which was very disconcerting given that I was puffing and panting through contraction after contraction.

As a rough estimate, the time between the start of established labour (4cm dilation) and full dilation (10cm) is 6 to 12 hours. This is for first time pregnancies only and any subsequent labours are usually a lot faster – just to make you feel better.

You may feel the urge to push quite early on but until your cervix is fully dilated you will be advised against it. You will be fully dilated when the baby's head can be seen popping out of your cervix. To stop the initial urge to push it may help to take short, sharp breaths, like little puffs. Imagine you are trying to quickly blow out the candles on a cake and you have the idea.

The heartbeat of your baby will be monitored throughout your labour to make sure baby is okay. Your midwife is watching for any changes. With my 3rd baby labour progressed really quickly and before I knew it I was pushing away. I noticed more and more people entering the room – about 6 or 7 in total – but was so caught up in the moment that I didn't fully understand until later that my labour was rushed as my baby had the cord wrapped around his throat. If your midwife says push with every ounce of strength you have, don't question her, just do it.

If all is going well, after some time you will all of a sudden have a massive urge to push. Let the midwife know so she can make sure everything is ready and then push with all your might.

If labour isn't progressing as quickly as it should be then your midwife may want to try speeding things up. If your waters haven't broken already then they will be broken for you during a vaginal examination. That may sound odd, as I was under the impression that waters breaking were one of the first signs of labour but remember that not all women are the same, and things don't always happen in the same way. You can go into labour without your waters breaking, and your labour can go on for several hours before your waters break, or you have your waters broken for you. Don't panic if this hasn't happened and just let the midwives know your situation so they can act accordingly.

If the waters being broken still doesn't speed things up then you may be given a hormone via a drip to encourage contractions. Not to be a big, fat meanie or anything, but if you have to be induced then usually you can count on labour being a lot more painful than if things go naturally. It can't be helped; if your body needs a push then it needs a push. Things work, things don't work, it's just the way it is unfortunately. There's no rhyme or reason to why one person has a quick labour and the other person doesn't. If you are induced and your birth plan was an "all-natural" plan then you may want to reconsider. However, as I've said several times throughout this book so far, every single person and every single delivery is different. Just because you are induced doesn't mean you will have to endure a 30 hour labour, your body may react to the drugs perfectly and you could be delivered within a few hours.

Second stage of labour – Birth
When your cervix is fully dilated the next stage is actually delivering your baby. Find a good position and get comfortable – if that is even possible. (It's not.) Some people like to kneel against the pillows, some people like to lie on their back and others find it easier to lie on their sides. Do whatever you find the easiest, whether that is standing up against the bed, or squatting on the bed. Lying on your side is probably the best position to take if you are feeling really tired, and is also a great position for your baby.

You will feel the need to push urgently. If you are fully dilated then you're ready to go, not long now! It may feel like you need a really massive poop. Push down hard, taking deep breaths as you do. You'll probably push a few times before the contraction ends and after each contraction you'll have to get ready for the next one. As the birth gets closer and closer so do your contractions until it feels almost as if they are sitting on top of each other. One will stop and seconds later it seems like the other is starting already.

Don't kid yourself, this is tough. And exhausting. Hear the end you will feel like you've had the longest and hardest workout of your life. You'll be sweaty and panting and if you have one moment of sanity you'll probably be thinking you must look an absolute wreck. You probably do, but at the same time you don't. Who gives a hoot what you look like, you're performing one of the most miraculous things anyone will ever witness, the birth of a human being. For some strange reason, as messy as you look, to your partner you will take on an almost angelic glow. You are having their child after all, and they can see how hard it is and through my experience, and the experience of all of my childbearing friends, the men find the whole thing amazing. This is the only moment that they will be in awe of you. You are amazing, messy hair and all.

This is also the part where your birthing partner comes into their own. Whilst your experiencing the worst pain of your life, if your birthing partner is worth their salt, they will calm you, reassure you, stroke your back and be exactly who you need them to be right then. There are no rules at this point, whatever works just go with it. If you need to shout abuse at him/her then go for it. I tried a scream, but was chastised by my midwife! Push, push and push some more. When you feel like you can push no more, you can and you will. At some point you may feel, and say, that you want to give up. I did. Each time. You won't give up though, it's simply impossible to do.

The birthing stage can take up to an hour, and it will feel like forever. Once the baby's head is visible you will be asked to slow your pushing down. You want your baby's head to be born slowly and gently to minimise any tearing. If it looks like you will tear you may be offered an episiotomy (a cut). Take it, you feel it much less than the tear and it seems to heal a lot better. I've had both and I would go with the episiotomy each time.

My first labour I had a cut, my second labour I had a tear. At the start of my third labour I told my midwife that if it came down to it I wanted the cut before I had the chance to tear. I don't know whether that is just my personal experience but I think it makes sense as the cut would be cleaner and much more controlled than any possible tearing.

Once your baby's head is out then the rest is relatively easy. Just one more push and the body is born, and literally minutes later the whole horrid mess feels like a century ago as you look down into your baby's face.

It may sound corny but just wait and see. The feelings that take over you cannot be described. That it makes grown men shed tears is nothing to the feeling of love and complete adoration you will experience. Never before will you have held something so precious and utterly dependent on you in your hands. The feeling is addictive, and it grows with each passing day – why do you think we have more when we emphatically state "no more" during the birth?

Before the cord is even cut your baby could be nestling in your arms. Your birthing partner has the option of cutting the cord, and John cut each of ours. It's one of those magical moments and for some strange reason, something the men seem to boast about. Guess they can't boast about much else during that time.

Don't be alarmed if your baby is covered in a creamy, slimy substance – that is what is called the vernix and it acted as protection in the uterus. Your baby may also have a bit of blood on them, but this again is absolutely normal.

The best way to immediately start the bonding process with your new bundle of wonderfulness is to initiate some skin-on-skin contact. You want your baby snuggled into your warm skin so they can feel the instant protection of their mummy. If the vernix and blood is freaking you out a bit you can ask your midwife to clean your baby up a little bit before you have a snuggle.

If you are not given your baby straightaway then try not to worry too much. If your baby is having trouble breathing or needs a quick check then the midwives and hospital staff will endeavour to carry out their work as quickly as possible so they can hand baby back as soon as they can.

Third stage of labour – Placenta

After your baby is born you then need to deliver the placenta. You will be offered an injection in your thigh to speed up delivery of the placenta. I had the injection each time and the placenta came out literally minutes later. It feels a bit weird, as you can feel the sac of fluid and other gunk sliding out. If you're interested, ask to have a quick look. It's fascinating as you can see the sac where your baby has spent the last 9 months of its life.

What Happens Next?

If possible, see if you can help your baby latch on as soon after the birth as possible. It will help with the breastfeeding process latr on and also helps your uterus to contract. Babies will start sucking almost immediately, although they won't last long. Just getting then to take your nipple in their mouth is enough as it just helps to start the breastfeeding process.

Even if you are not planning on breastfeeding it is advised that you try to do this. If you can breastfeed for even the first few days you will hae given your baby a fantastic start in life.

In England it is general practice to keep you in hospital for at least 5 hours after the birth. This is to make sure that everything is okay and no complications suddenly develop. The midwives would prefer to see baby feed and wee before they are comfortable allowing you both to go home. They'll take a note of the exact weight of your baby and put a little band on their ankles and/or wrists for identification purposes.

You will be offered a vitamin K injection, which is the most effective way of preventing a rare bleeding disorder known as haemorrhagic disease of the newborn. If you would prefer you can opt for oral doses but I haven't had any problem with the injection. All 3 of mine had it and I experienced absolutely no side effects whatsoever.

While you're holding your baby, if you had an episiotomy or tore you will be stitched up. If you only had a small tear then you will not be stitched and the tear will be left to heal naturally. You will be given a local anaesthetic while they stitch you up, but it's not the most comfortable feeling in the world.

Before leaving the hospital you will also be given the chance to have a bath or shower. If you are lucky you will have your own personal shower room – I loved this with my 3rd child. With my 1st and 2nd child I had to use a communal bathroom, but the midwives ensure that the rooms are clean and even run the bath for you. You may have a bit of difficulty getting into the bath and you will definitely feel sore and tender so it's best if your birthing partner can help you.

Don't be concerned if you see quite a bit of blood running down your leg as you're showering. You will have to wear thick pads for anything upto 2 weeks after giving birth as you will continue to lose blood as your body gets back to normal. If you are concerned about the amount of blood you are losing then ask your midwife or health visitor straightaway. They will be more than happy to check that everything is okay.

Did You Know?

Around 1 in 8 women have an assisted birth, where forceps or a ventouse are used to help get the baby out.

Summary

In this section we talked mainly about me, my favourite topic. I never tire of telling my labour stories, and you probably won't either. They define you and they become the key pivotal moments of your life. Before kids we had fun, sure, but we didn't have the purpose of life that having kids brings. The stories of how they got here in the first place are special, and should be cherished as they make us who we are.

Even at the grand old age of 36 I still like to know that my mum remembers the time I was born and how long her labour took with me. I take a secret pleasure in hearing her recount stories of me when I was a tiny baby (and apparently a not very nice one at that, something about a LOT of crying). Your children will probably take the same pleasure in hearing you talk about them as babies, and even if they don't it will still make you smile when you remember how things were.

Hopefully this section of the book didn't scare you too much. Whilst labour is hard, and extremely painful for most, we keep on doing it, and that should tell you something. If I'd been that traumatized by the whole event I wouldn't have had another. It's one day, or if you're unlucky two, and then you spend the rest of your life loving this tiny little human who grew inside you and needed and loved you even when no-one else did. There are no words to describe that first moment you finally meet them.

You'll remember the pain, but there'll come a point when you just don't care. Think about how you want the birth to go, visit the hospitals in your area and decide what kind of birth you want to have. Meet regularly with your midwife or doctor and discuss options and air any worries you may have. When the big day comes try not to get too flustered and make sure you have a birthing partner who will be with you every step of the way.

It may not feel like it when you're going through it, but you can and will do it. The fun starts once you're home.

6 THE FOURTH TRIMESTER

I love the whole idea of the fourth trimester. The fourth trimester is supposed to be more like the time your baby spent inside your womb rather than the time they will spend outside of it.

The term was introduced by Dr Karp, who determined that a baby needs nothing more than the almost constant attention of its mother to help it adapt to life outside of the womb. It all comes down to the fact that whilst most mammal babies are able to move around on their own quite quickly after birth, human babies are much more reliant on their parents and are not ready to face the world for a much longer time.

Apparently, as humans adapted and evolved, our pelvises became smaller meaning that we effectively shortened the time we could carry a baby through pregnancy as the head would be too big if it stayed inside for much longer. The premise of the fourth trimester then is that babies are born 3 months too early and it is because of this that we should try and keep their outside world as close to their inside world as we can.

Sounds crazy doesn't it? But then think about... Imagine you have been living in the safest environment known to man for the whole of your life. It's quiet, there are noises but they're muffled and aren't a threat at all. You have constant food and drink and can wake and sleep whenever you want. You feel as if you are being rocked back and forth in a comforting caress for most of the day and are cocooned inside a warm, gooey substance.

All of a sudden you are thrust into an alien world of lights and noise and constant change. You have no access to food, you are cold and dry, you are left alone lying on a flat surface with no movement and the warm, safe environment you loved so much has gone. Put that way we can see how stressful it must be being a newborn. Imagine the process in which they learn that crying means they potentially get what they want, be that food, a clean nappy or a loving cuddle.

Forget what you read about babies being manipulative and needing to be trained as soon as possible. Forget all this nonsense about cry-down sleeping and controlled routines. Forget this notion that babies should go to bed at 6pm and not wake up until 7am. It's all westernised rubbish designed to make us think that we are more important than anyone else, including our own child, and that we should quite literally cast baby aside and get on with earning money and doing what we want to do.

Want to know the easiest and most rewarding way to make certain your baby is happy? Give him/her the love and attention that they so desperately need. Only in the West do we think it's acceptable to allow a baby to cry until he/she falls asleep.

I love the concept of the fourth trimester (yes I know I've already said this, but I just do!). I love the notion that we should hold our babies as much as we can in those first 3 months, and beyond. I love the notion that it is more than normal that our babies should wake every few hours or less. I love the notion that if your baby wants to fall asleep whilst feeding he/she can and you won't be saddled with a bad habit for the rest of their lives.

We are told that we should try and get our lives back to normal and reclaim our sleeping rituals, but if you think of the size of a baby's stomach it should make sense that they have to refill it much more often than you and I do, given that it's so tiny to begin with. We are told that sleep should never follow feeding as this will instill bad habits that will refuse to be shaken. Babies can't learn bad habits, and they certainly can't learn them at 3 months of age.

So what should we be doing? Without knowing what I was doing I pretty much followed the fourth trimester guidelines. I just couldn't put my kids down, they were just so cute and loved having cuddles and I loved cuddling them.

When I had Jack, because he was so tiny and had come so early he needed feeding almost hourly. Jack was a really clingy baby and would cry whenever I put him down. It was nigh on impossible to keep the house clean, and in the end I simply kept the house semi-presentable and shied away from the maintenance side of things.

If you are going to follow the principles of the fourth trimester then you really need to agree the process with your partner to make sure they are on board. If they come home from a long day at work and the house is a tip or the tea isn't cooked because you spent the day appeasing a crying or sickly baby, then they need to be able to set aside any grievances and understand that you were dealing with your baby first.

This isn't an excuse for doing nothing but sitting and watching tv whilst giving baby a cuddle. You can still get around and get things done. Invest in a good baby carrier and carry your baby with you wherever you go.

I swore by my baby carrier with my first child. I used it every single day and John loved going for walks with Jack strapped against his chest. Using a baby carrier is a great way to encourage the bond between father and son/daughter. They get to feel the closeness you feel when holding your baby close, and get to experience some of the magic.

There are some fantastic baby carriers on the market right now and the choices are vast. You can choose between the more conventional Baby Bjorn carrier, an Ergobaby soft-structured carrier, a baby sling or the current carrier of choice the baby wrap.

They may look a bit intimidating due to the amount of fabric but the baby wrap would be my baby carrier of choice for the first few months, especially if you want to fully embrace the fourth trimester concept of keeping baby close at all times.

Using a baby carrier will allow you to have your hands free whilst your baby is attached to your front, snuggled up to your chest. They love being so close and take comfort from hearing your heart, something which they used to be able to do constantly whilst in your womb. Did you know that whilst your baby spent 100% of their time feeling close to you before being born, on average they only spend 40% of their time close to you once born? What a massive change they have to go through.

Sleep

For me, sleep ties in with feeding. I committed the cardinal sin (apparently) of allowing my baby to feed and then fall asleep whilst feeding. Apparently, according to most medical advice, this is the wrong thing to do as you are encouraging your baby to develop bad habits and to need to feed to get to sleep.

If you agree then forgive me for airing my judgement but I did it with each child, each child fed on demand and slept when they fell asleep. I fed them during the night when they woke up and fed them first thing in the morning when I was still waking up.

In the first 3 months I pretty much kept each baby close by throughout the night. In the evening I would keep the moses basket close by, usually in the same room or in the adjacent room so I could listen out for any grumbles. When I went to bed I'd put the moses basket right next to my bed on the stand and when my baby woke up I would bring him into bed with me.

Probably the most controversial opinion I will share in this book is the co-sleeping one. I co-slept with each of my children. With my first child I really tried to keep him in the moses basket but every time I got him back to sleep and went to lay him down in his basket he would wake up, and then I would start feeding again so he would fall asleep. I would try to keep him from making too much noise as I didn't want to wake the hubby so would pick him up almost immediately after he started to cry. He fall back asleep in my arms pretty easily, snuggled up against me, but as soon as I tried to lay him down he would wake.

Eventually, after doing this 5 or 6 times every night I was so exhausted that I would often find myself dozing off to sleep with my baby lying in my arms and me half propped up against the pillows. I'd drift off to sleep while I was still holding Jack and then jump awake shortly after, worried about falling asleep and potentially losing my grip on my son.

It was after a few consecutive nights of no sleep that one night I gave in and lay down and had Jack lie next to me. He fell asleep quickly and I did the same. I made sure the cover was away from him and I put his own little blanket over him. I made sure he had lots of room at the side of him so he couldn't roll over and fall out – not that he could roll! He slept better than he had ever slept that first time I tried co-sleeping, and so did I. And that was it, I had found a potential way out of the never-ending lack of sleep.

I would still put Jack down in his moses basket, and later on in his cot, and would try to put him down when he woke the first couple of times, but by about 4am Jack would always be in our bed. And it was exactly the same for the other two.

At first the hubby wasn't too bothered as he could see that I was getting some sleep finally and thus was more inclined to do stuff in the day. After a few weeks though, he started expressing his annoyance at having to share his bed with a baby. I did try to get Jack to sleep by himself but he just wanted to be close to me, he'd even put his legs against mine and make sure either his feet or his arms were touching me. I secretly loved the feel of my baby nestled up against me and sleeping soundly and happily. The husband couldn't say the same.

We ended up having a few arguments about it but he was unable or unwilling to help with the sleep situation. One night though, it was John who was sleeping in bed, and I had got up to use the toilet. Jack stirred, looking for the warmth of my touch but I wasn't there. John was though, and pulled Jack in close. Of course Jack snuggled right in and went back to sleep. I think it was that moment that John realised why I liked co-sleeping so much.

It may not be everyone's cup of tea and I have the upmost respect for the people who can stick to their guns and see through the tough times and get their baby sleeping soundly in their own bed, in their own room. I have to admit though; it's just not for me. Maybe I'm lazy and find it easier allowing my baby to sleep with me. Whatever you may think, it works for me. It works for my husband, and more importantly, it works for my baby.

I'm not advocating you do the same, and if you do decide to give it a go, research the best ways to do it. Read up on how you can do it safely and with the minimum amount of risk for your baby. You do not want to be covering your baby with your covers, particularly if they are duvet covers, as these are too heavy. You can't let your baby get his/her head covered with blankets, you can't let them get too hot, and you can't let them get too close to the edge and fall off. Be careful. Be safe. Do NOT drink alcohol or take anything which would impair your reaction times or increase your drowsiness. The worst possible scenario you could face is waking up to find you have rolled over onto your sleeping baby and cut off his air supply.

If you play it safe and take all the precautions necessary then co-sleeping can be a really beneficial way for both you and your baby to get the sleep you need. If you have exhausted all other avenues, have found yourself falling asleep on the couch or a chair with baby in your arms – a lot more dangerous than sharing a bed – or just simply need to get some rest, I would suggest giving it a try. To make sure you are doing it safely head on over to the internet. Sites such as www.attachmentparenting.org and Dr.

James McKenna's Mother Baby Sleep Laboratory site, http://cosleeping.nd.edu will give you advice on the correct way to co-sleep. If you're wondering who Dr. James McKenna is he is one of the leading voices on the benefits of co-sleeping.

Of course it's up to you how you deal with bedtime and we all have our preferences. I'm not about to preach about the right way and the wrong way, mainly because I'm not suitably experienced to do so. I'm simply sharing my experiences and my choices. My idea of bedtime contrasts massively with how bedtime actually goes down in our house. I had visions of implementing a routine early on and sticking to it rigidly and of having children who took themselves off to bed once I called out "bedtime". The scary part of that scenario is that there are apparently children who do just that! I can't pretend that I wouldn't love it if mine did, but they don't. 10 minutes of cajoling leads to 15 minutes of getting ready for bed, progressing to 20 minutes of stories, 5 minutes of tucking in and cuddles and about 50 minutes of revisiting the bedroom every so often to quiet them down or carry them back to bed. On a good day I can be done in 25 minutes, on a bad day it can take closer to 2 hours. Yep, I really don't have this bedtime thing down to a fine art at all, or any kind of art if you want to be blunt. So probably not the best person to follow for advice then!?

Feeding

Tied into sleeping, purely because in the first few weeks everything is tied into sleeping, given that that is all babies seem to do, is feeding. I fed on demand, which is when you allow your baby to tell you when they want feeding.

If you are breastfeeding then feeding on demand is the easiest thing to do. Simply lift up your top, flick down the fastener on your nursing bra and off you go. If you're worried about feeding outside the home then take a blanket or oversized muslin or scarf with you and use that to discreetly cover up the top half of your body.

I'm pretty good at this bit. I even considered training to be a breastfeeding helper. I thought I'd never get the hang of it that first time but by baby number 3 I had him latched on within seconds and I've never looked back.

I'm not going to get all preachy, heck, why not, it's not like I've held back before… breastfeeding is best. We all know it. Maybe we like to think formula is just as good, but really!? Of course it isn't. I know people have their reasons, but I can't praise breastfeeding enough. I know parents who've bottle fed their children who have gone through lots of bowel issues with them. I think it may have something to do with the milk. As a general rule, the numbers of issues babies have with pooping when breastfed is a lot less to those who are bottle fed.

And that's only a tiny reason to breastfeed. Your body contains all the nutrition a baby could ever want. To top that it also contains antibodies that help fight infection. And there's another statistic for you, the number of babies suffering from illnesses is less in breastfed babies than in bottle fed babies.

Breastfed babies tend not to be so heavy and are generally not overfed. They are healthier because they are getting exactly what they need from you. Another great reason for breastfeeding is the fact that it is so cheap – it costs zilch – and is pretty much on tap – whip your boob out and you're ready to go.

Bottle feed if you so desire, but please please please just give breastfeeding a go. If you only do it for a few days then you will have done your bit and passed on some much-needed goodness to your little one.

Summary

In summary then, the fourth trimester is all about:
- ➢ Keeping your baby close
- ➢ Co-sleeping when necessary
- ➢ Baby wearing
- ➢ Giving up on the notion of returning to old sleeping habits
- ➢ Feeding on demand
- ➢ Breastfeeding if possible
- ➢ Lots of cuddles and snuggles
- ➢ Forget about creating "bad" habits, it's just not going to happen

7 CONCLUSION

I hope you've enjoyed reading through this book and have picked up some hints and tips along the way. We've gone from getting pregnant right through to the labour and first few weeks and I hope that sharing my own personal experiences has brought the factual parts to life a bit more. Whilst I've emphasised the rollercoaster journey you're embarking on, it is nothing to the rollercoaster of emotions you will experience as a parent. It really is true that life means so much more with children in the picture, you will love them more than you ever thought possible, and at the same time they will drive you crazy with their endless chattering and potty training escapades, but like me, you probably wouldn't miss a moment. Notice the word "probably" I stuck in there?

I always say to my husband that it is easier going to work than it is staying at home with the kids, and I fully believe that. I went back to work after my first 2 children, and whilst it was heart wrenching to leave them, getting to drink a cup of tea while it was still hot was a novelty. Eating lunch without it being pinched or going cold was a luxury I still enjoy every now and again.

Enjoy the time you have with your babies, however long that may be, and enjoy the feeling of being pregnant. You are a walking miracle. Make sure you remind yourself of that when you start feeling down and fat and miserable – you will at some point! Drum into your partner how important it is for them to be supportive and how much your lives are going to change once your bundle of joy appears.

If you have any concerns during pregnancy or after the birth then please do not hesitate to contact your local doctor as they will be able to help. It doesn't matter how trivial or stupid you feel, if you are even slightly concerned it's better to just ask and check. A good doctor would prefer you to ask rather than adopt a wait and see attitude and only seek their advice when it's too late to use preventative remedies.

I realise it's a bit of a mish mash of advice, silly stories and annoying lecturing. I set out writing this with the aim of not appearing to be judgmental or not trying to push my own beliefs on others, and I think I pretty much failed catastrophically on that. However, I do hope you found it an interesting read and laughed at least once.

What I hope you got out of it most is that everyone walks into motherhood knowing not much of anything, and then suddenly we become the masters of it, proffering advice to whomever will listen. If you're scared now just give it a few months and you will feel like you've been doing it forever. You will forget what your old life was like and will never want to give up what you are about to receive – a love so strong it will take your breath away and bring a tear to your eye at a moment's notice.

Enjoy your pregnancy, and look forward to what is bound to be the most exciting, life changing, life defining, exhausting and chaotic ride of your whole existence.

ABOUT THE AUTHOR

Gracie Little is the mother to 3 energetic boys, all under the age of 6 at the writing of this book. Gracie, likes most mothers, loves learning about her little men and would love the whole process of childrearing and motherhood to be a lot more intuitive and a lot less formal. She wrote this book to demonstrate that there are women out there who are doing what they feel right rather than what they are told, and it is working. Her hopes for this book is simply that it helps someone to feel that they are not alone and that, although they may feel run down and tired and incapable of coping, that a lot of women feel the same way and none of us are perfect all of the time.

"Get messy, muck about and most of all have fun" is her motto.